B362.1 KOS.

362.1 KOG (B)

DATE DUE

26/6/00			
2/3/01			
11/6/02			
22/9/03			
GAYLORD			PRINTED IN U.S.A.

Making Use of Clinical Audit

Health Services Management

Series Editors:
Chris Ham, Health Services Management Centre, University of Birmingham
Chris Heginbotham, The Riverside Mental Health Trust, London

The British National Health Service is one of the biggest and most complex organizations in the developed world. Employing around one million people and accounting for £36 billion of public expenditure, the Service is of major concern to both the public and politicians. Management within the NHS faces a series of challenges in ensuring that resources are deployed efficiently and effectively. These challenges include the planning and management of human resources, the integration of professionals into the management process, and making sure that services meet the needs of patients and the public.

Against this background, the Health Services Management series addresses the many issues and practical problems faced by people in managerial roles in health services.

Current and forthcoming titles

Justin Keen (ed.): *Information Management in Health Services*
John Øvretveit: *Purchasing for Health*
Richard Joss and Maurice Kogan: *Advancing Quality: Total Quality Management in the National Health Service*
Maurice Kogan and Sally Redfern *et al.*: *Making Use of Clinical Audit: A guide to practice in the health professions*
Steve Harrison: *Managing Health Services: A basic text*
Judith Allsop and Linda Mulcahy: *Risk Management in Medical Settings*
Valerie Iles: *Real Managers in Healthcare Organizations*
Gordon Marnoch: *Doctors and Management in the National Health Service*

Making Use of Clinical Audit

A guide to practice in the health professions

Maurice Kogan and Sally Redfern

with Anémone Kober, Ian Norman,
Tim Packwood and Sarah Robinson

Open University Press
Buckingham · Philadelphia

Open University Press
Celtic Court
22 Ballmoor
Buckingham
MK18 1XW

and

1900 Frost Road, Suite 101
Bristol, PA 19007, USA

First Published 1995

A catalogue record of this book is available from the British Library

ISBN   0 335 19542 3 (pb)   0 335 19543 1 (hb)

Library of Congress Cataloging-in-Publication Data
Making use of clinical audit: a guide to practice in the health
   professions / by Maurice Kogan and Sally Redfern; with Anémone
   Kober . . . [et al.].
        p.   cm. — (Health services management series)
   Includes bibliographical references and index.
   ISBN 0–335–19543–1 (hb). — ISBN 0–335–19542–3 (pb)
   1. Medical care—Great Britain—Evaluation. 2. Medical audit—
Great Britain. I. Kogan, Maurice. II. Redfern, Sally J.
III. Kober, Anémone, 1962– . IV. Series: Health services
management.
   [DNLM: 1. Quality Assurance, Health Care—organization &
administration—Great Britain. W 84 FA1 M2 1995]
RA399.G7M35   1995
362.1'068'5—dc20
DNLM/DLC
for Library of Congress   95–10765
                                                                          CIP

Typeset by Graphicraft Typesetters Ltd, Hong Kong
Printed in Great Britain by Biddles Ltd, Guildford and King's Lynn

Contents

The authors

Maurice Kogan, Professor of Government and Social Administration and Joint Director, Centre for the Evaluation of Public Policy and Practice, Brunel University, where he has been the Head of the Department of Government, Dean of the Faculty of Social Sciences and Acting Vice-Chancellor. He has published extensively in the policies and organization of the health service, education and higher education, social services and science policy.

Sally Redfern, Professor of Nursing and Director, Nursing Research Unit, King's College, London University. Her research and publications are concerned with care of elderly people and quality assessment and evaluation of nursing services.

Dr Anémone Kober, formerly Research Associate, Nursing Research Unit, King's College, London University, now Maître de Conférences, Université de Paris III.

Dr Ian Norman, Senior Lecturer, Department of Nursing Studies, King's College, London University.

Tim Packwood, Senior Lecturer, Department of Government, Brunel University.

Sarah Robinson, Senior Research Fellow, Nursing Research Unit, King's College, London University.

Preface

The quality issue is everywhere in the National Health Service and many committed and knowledgeable groups and individuals are working to make sense of its complexities. Yet those anxious to improve quality find it difficult to identify useful definitions of it, particularly since its components legitimately differ in different fields of work and at different levels of complex systems.

This book is intended to help all of those in the health service, and those working in similar fields of social and other care, to take the initiative in establishing quality assurance in their areas of work. It is particularly directed to elucidating and developing those forms of quality assurance defined as clinical audit.

We owe many debts of gratitude to those associated with the project forming the basis for this book. In 1992, the NHS Executive invited the Centre for the Evaluation of Public Policy and Practice (CEPPP) at Brunel University and the Nursing Research Unit (NRU) at King's College, University of London to conduct a project on clinical audit in the therapy professions. The professions for study chosen by our Department of Health 'customers' had been the subject of a pioneering report by Professor Charles Normand and colleagues (Normand et al. 1991a, 1991b). This had advocated a common framework for audit in clinical psychology, occupational therapy, physiotherapy and speech and language therapy. Obviously, all of the other health professions had claims to be included in Normand's and our study; we are confident that this book will prove relevant to the concerns of the whole range of clinical occupations within the health fields.

The NHS Executive asked us to establish a range of good practice for clinical audit in the therapy professions. This was to involve 'investigating known examples of good practice, disaggregating the principles of components of each model, and then disseminating those models, perhaps reaggregating them on the way'.

We could only undertake our project through collaboration with the four professions to develop and evaluate a set of models on which their audit activities could be based. Whilst we looked for commonalities between them we aimed to extend the range of choice available to the professions rather than to create prescriptive patterns.

We therefore depended largely upon contact with those knowledgeable in the professional field. We took up nine cases of multi- and uni-professional clinical audit activity in a range of the professions and in a geographical spread throughout England. Throughout, because our intention was not to produce models derived from abstract theories about professional practice or ways of evaluating or auditing them, we worked closely with those active in the fields. The models that have emerged are thus based on the views, experiences and judgements of experts within the four professions. We thank all the providers and purchasers we met, particularly members of the four professions, for giving us so much information, time and patience.

This study was funded by the Department of Health. We are grateful to successive members of the 'customer' divisions of the NHS Executive and to members of the Research and Development Division of the Department for their support and critique throughout the inception and completion of the project. We are particularly grateful to Sheelagh Richards, Occupational Therapy Officer at the Department, for support throughout.

In all of this, the contribution of our expert advisory group has been indispensable. Its members are listed in Appendix 1.

This book is the result of work undertaken cooperatively by members of the Centre for the Evaluation of Public Policy and Practice at Brunel University and the Nursing Research Unit at King's College London. All members of the joint team contributed to all parts of it but each of us took responsibility for drafting individual chapters, and the views expressed in this publication are those of the authors and not necessarily those of the Department of Health.

This book was collated and edited from the official report on our project made to the Department of Health. The chapters and appendices are attributed to those who were the main sources of the material edited. This is necessary because of the general demands made on academics to demonstrate their research outcomes.

The fieldwork was undertaken by all members of the team but on a full-time basis by Dr Anémone Kober, the project research associate, who also contributed fully to the team effort of conceptualization and writing-up throughout the project.

In Chapter 1, we define some of the terms essential to an understanding of clinical audit, and offer an account of the changing meanings of quality, quality assurance, quality improvement and clinical audit itself.

In Chapter 2 we sketch in the policy background and establish the relationship between clinical audit and other forms of quality assurance and knowledge generation.

In Chapter 3 we enter into a detailed analysis of the components and sequence of clinical audit. Is it cyclical in nature or are there other linear or non-linear sequences? How does the clinical audit cycle connect with the patient care, standards setting and change cycles?

Chapter 4 provides a detailed account of clinical audit and the progress it has made in the four professions. It clarifies the different modes of clinical audit, takes up the issue of outcome analysis, and discusses multi-disciplinarity. It considers how far clinical audit is affected by contextual factors.

Chapter 5 identifies the benefits of clinical audit and the constraints experienced in achieving it. Chapter 6 locates clinical audit within the management of health care systems. And in Chapter 7 we work through our materials and arguments in order to offer ways forward and to suggest the components of effective modelling of clinical audit.

Glossary

broad definition of audit the entire audit (or quality assurance) cycle including measurement and change in practice when indicated.

BS5750 a registration process in which set quality assurance systems are inspected and validated, on criteria set by the organization, by inspectors from the British Standards Institute.

closely associated clinical audit assessment of activities closely associated to core clinical practice.

core clinical audit assessment of clinical activities directly related to patients, often involving technical activities.

generic quality the common aspects of quality in the way that work is organized and managed, its results and relationships as applied by whole services or management units.

King's Fund organizational audit an accreditation scheme concentrating on the quality of organizational arrangements.

less closely associated clinical audit assessment of activities less closely associated to core clinical practice.

outcome the health, well-being or other state of the patient or client including the change in status attributable to antecedent care.

Patient's Charter the Patient's Charter states patients' rights to access to all quality of care. It requires health authorities to make returns to the Department of Health on the extent to which certain national objectives, e.g. reduction of waiting lists, have been achieved.

process the complex of interactions, transactions and activities between health care workers and their patients or clients.

resource management initiative was designed 'to enable the NHS to give a better service . . . by helping clinicians and other managers to make more informed judgements about how the resources they control can be used to maximum effect'.

restricted definition of audit the measurement stage within the audit (or quality assurance) cycle.

structure organizational factors that determine the conditions under which care is given, e.g. the physical environment, management style, staffing levels, support services.

systemic quality the quality of a comprehensive and integrated set of services to meet the health needs of a local population, as applied by whole services or management units.

technical quality the specialist quality of processes of care applied by individual providers in their work.

total quality management an advanced and integrated, corporately led programme of organizational change designed to create a culture of continuous improvement based on customer-orientated definitions of quality. It also entails staff empowerment and systemic monitoring and evaluation of quality.

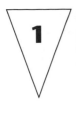

1 What is audit?

Ian Norman and Sally Redfern

We begin with a few essential definitions, to be explained more fully as we go along. First of all, what is audit? Audit is a word that has acquired different meanings. It has been defined in a specific sense as assessing or measuring quality of care. It is often used, though, more broadly, as measuring quality *and* changing practice when improvement to care or treatment is required.

We discuss audit and clinical audit in some detail later in this chapter. First, though, we set clinical audit within the framework of quality and quality assurance in health care. The chapter moves from the concept of quality, to quality assurance and then to audit and clinical audit. We convey therapists' understanding of clinical audit and their progress in developing audit activities in their professions. In the final section of this chapter we discuss the challenges of outcome measurement. In Chapter 4, we give examples of progress made by the therapy professions to assess the outcomes of their care and treatment and to move from patient care outcome assessment to assessment of service outcomes.

Quality

Our aim in these discussions is to show where concepts of audit come from and the extent to which they vary over time and different work and social settings. This information forms a basis to the more practical guidance for professionals and managers seeking to install or improve audit that follows in later chapters. The literature is voluminous and wide ranging but what is striking is the inconsistency in the way common terms are used. This confusion in terminology may have followed the burgeoning interest in quality, quality assurance and audit, as a result of which a number of terms have become current before their meaning is clear (Whittington and Finlay 1991). Or the meaning of terms and labels to describe and define quality may reflect the prevailing states of power, authority and autonomy of different professional groups (Pollitt 1992).

The notion of quality is elusive and dynamic. Elusive because definition depends on value judgements by individuals and society. Dynamic because definitions of quality change over time to reflect current social values of health, and expectations of professional–client relationships and health services.

We focus here on *operational* definitions, which take the form of specific statements to be used in practice. Crosby (1989), for example, defines high quality as 'zero deficits' and Juran (1988) as 'fitness for use'. Juran's focus is on products or services that meet the needs of customers and increase their satisfaction. Operational definitions of quality often incorporate a consideration of cost; for example, high quality is the capacity of a product to fulfil its intended purpose at the least possible cost (Feigenbaum 1951).

In health care, operational definitions of quality reflect the importance of actual care conforming to pre-set criteria (Donabedian 1970). Whether cost should be included as part of the definition is more controversial, although it is certainly a major consideration in countries, such as the USA, with insurance-funded health care provision. Concern over cost has increased in the UK as health reforms seek to generate improvements through the creation of internal markets (Secretaries of State for Health 1989).

If we are to evaluate the degree of conformity between care given and pre-set criteria, the definition of quality must include clearly articulated standards and criteria. Donabedian (1988b, 1988c) distinguishes between maximum and optimum standards of care. Maximum standards ignore cost and define highest quality care as that which is expected to achieve the greatest possible improvement in health. Optimum standards exclude care that is disproportionately expensive in terms of expected health gain.

We now turn to a more detailed consideration of health care quality by looking at the work of two authorities in the field, Donabedian and Maxwell.

Donabedian's components of health care quality and framework for quality assessment

Much of the early work on defining health care quality was by Donabedian, who describes three components relevant to health care (Donabedian 1980):

- *goodness of technical care* refers to the effectiveness of health care, its ability to achieve the greatest improvement in health status possible within the conventional wisdom of medicine, that is, of science, technology and clinical skills

- *goodness of interpersonal relationships* amongst those involved in health care, in particular the relationship between the user (patient) and the provider (therapist, nurse, doctor, other health care professional). Thus, an important aspect of high quality care is that patients be treated with respect and their autonomy and interests safeguarded
- *goodness of amenities*, which refers to creature comforts and aesthetic attributes of the health care setting. These can be difficult to distinguish from interpersonal care because privacy, courtesy, acceptability, comfort, promptness and so on are relevant to amenities as well as to interpersonal relationships. Donabedian emphasizes the inextricable intertwining of his components, thus demonstrating his appreciation of quality as a whole entity.

He describes four definitions of quality of medical care:

- his *individualized* definition judges quality with reference to patients' values, means, wishes and expectations
- his *social* definition recognizes that there must be a net benefit for the population and effective social distribution of that benefit
- his *absolutist* definition requires care to achieve an optimum balance between health risks and benefits, and relates closely to scientific and technical aspects of medicine; thus, useless or redundant care is equivalent to poor care because it wastes money and resources
- his last definition specifies that the 'primary function of medical care is to advance the patient's welfare' (Donabedian 1980). This definition emphasizes patients as the judge of their own welfare and the importance of patient and doctor sharing the responsibility for balancing risks and benefits and defining objectives.

Although most of Donabedian's writings refer to medical care, his ideas are relevant to the work of all health care professionals.

Donabedian is probably best known for his application of a *systems-based* framework, referred to as *structure-process-outcome*, to inputs, processes and outputs of health care:

- *structure* refers to organizational factors that determine the conditions under which care is given, e.g. the physical environment, management style, staffing levels, support services
- *process* focuses upon the complex of interactions, transactions and activities between health care workers and their patients
- *outcome* is 'not simply a measure of health, well-being or any other state. Rather it is a change in status confidently attributable to antecedent care' (Donabedian 1988a). This definition highlights the importance of linking outcome to process and also reflects Donabedian's preference for a broad definition of health; outcomes can reflect improvements in social and psychological function as well as physical and psychological aspects.

Donabedian was successful in translating the elements of quality into an operational framework. This revolutionized methods for evaluating the quality of care and provided a powerful stimulus towards promoting a widespread, explicit concern for health care quality. In Chapter 4 we draw upon his framework in classifying audit activities.

According to Donabedian (1988a), the nature of the question asked and pragmatic constraints (e.g. availability of information, accuracy of measurement and cost) should determine the choice of whether to assess structure, process or outcome, or a combination. For example, outcome measurement alone will determine what good we are doing (Donabedian 1969). But if outcomes 'provide indirect evidence of whether the antecedent process corresponds to what is known or presumed to be the most efficacious care' (Donabedian 1988a) then outcome cannot be assessed independently of process. As a general rule Donabedian suggests that aspects of all three elements should be assessed.

Maxwell's elements of health care quality

One of the best-known developments of Donabedian's ideas in the UK is by Maxwell (1984), who puts forward six elements as a means of describing and measuring the quality of health care:

- *relevance*: the service or procedure is required by the individual or population
- *accessibility*: time, distance and structural access are within accepted norms
- *effectiveness*: the service achieves proper benefit for the individual or population
- *acceptability*: reasonable expectations of the patients and community are met
- *efficiency*: resources are well used
- *equity*: there is a fair share for all the community.

Maxwell maintains that each element should be recognized separately. Different methods of assessment are required for each and an acceptable level or standard would have to be agreed.

Later, he reports that the Audit Commission amalgamated his access and equity elements on the grounds that most inequalities are about uneven access (Maxwell 1992). Maxwell disagrees with this argument because there can be inequities which are unrelated to access – for example, possible prejudice and bias against ethnic minorities. He also points out that a multidimensional concept of quality, the flavour of the components and of policy trade-offs amongst them, is more important than the number of concepts involved.

Maxwell's (1992) combination of structure, process and outcome with his six elements of quality might be applied to any health care system to

	Structure	Process	Outcome
Efficiency	Avoid extravagance in structure, equipment, staffing	Throughput, staffing etc. Admission and discharge arrangements	Costs for comparable cases
Access		How many patients suitable for admission have to be refused because the unit is full?	What happens to patients refused or delayed admission because the unit is full?
Equity		Is there any evidence of bias in who is admitted and how they are treated?	Is there any evidence of bias in outcome?

Figure 1.1 Extract from Maxwell's quality assessment framework (From Maxwell 1992)

identify which aspects of performance are inadequately covered and require attention. Figure 1.1 shows an example using three of his elements.

Maxwell argues that this sort of framework is preferable for quality assessment compared to the NHS's allegiance to a mass of performance indicators whose purpose and relative importance are unclear.

Industrial models and modes of health care quality

Towards industrial models of quality in health care

Donabedian's structure-process-outcome framework has been interpreted as an inspection-based approach to quality evaluation (Harvey 1991) although this is not necessarily what Donabedian intended. Consequently, the early quality implementation programmes emphasized accreditation of structure, process and outcome standards by outside agencies. A prominent example is the Joint Commission for the Accreditation of Health Care Organizations (JCAHCO) in the USA. Another, in the UK, is the King's Fund Organizational Audit, which was introduced as a formal accreditation system of health care services. So far accreditation schemes are voluntary in this country but achieving accreditation standards is likely to become more important in the current competitive health care market.

A marked shift is discernible over the last few years in health care away from inspection-based models of quality assurance towards more proactive, prevention-orientated approaches derived from industrial models of quality based on a continuous quality improvement philosophy. Our view is that this has occurred because of growing concern about the lack of impact of quality improvement programmes on health care services. Attention is

rarely given to problems encountered when implementing actions for improvement. The efforts required to promote change receive only cursory
attention in medical audit (Maxwell 1992), and it is not unusual to find
that peer review groups resist having to collect data necessary to monitor
whether improvements are taking place (Freeling and Burton 1986). This
movement towards an industrial model of continuous quality improvement
is evident in the JCAHCO (O'Leary 1991) and also in the UK. Department
of Health funding established 17 total quality management pilot sites which
were evaluated by Brunel University (Joss *et al.* 1994; Joss and Kogan
1995).

Donabedian's conception of health care quality sits somewhat uneasily
with industrial quality models. His emphasis on the doctor– (or therapist–)
patient relationship tends to neglect the ways in which many others relate
to the patient and contribute to health care outcomes. The philosophy of
continuous quality improvement emphasizes these other contributions and
implies that the health care professional is almost always dependent upon
them for effective performance.

Following Donabedian, therapists can feel reassured that their patient
care is of high quality if they do their best within the current conventional
wisdom of the profession, whether or not their actions can be shown to
have beneficial results (outcomes). But this definition of quality does not
fit comfortably with total quality management's emphasis on value for
money which would hold that a service that does not meet clients' needs
would be in error, even if the input resources and processes are themselves
of high quality (Joss *et al.* 1994).

Donabedian (1993) acknowledges the value to health care of industrial
models of quality improvement in that they focus unequivocally on customers. This approach extends responsibility for quality throughout the
organization and, in so doing, it increases managers' responsibility and the
importance of understanding systems and processes. Donabedian does warn,
though, that attempts simply to apply industrial quality models to health
care may lead to increased emphasis on efficiency at the cost of clinical effectiveness and may underestimate the complexity of the client–practitioner
relationship.

Modes of health care quality

We follow the formulation proposed in the NHS total quality management
project (Joss *et al.* 1994; Joss and Kogan 1995) of three modes of quality
which can be regarded as central to improvement in the NHS and other
public services:

- *technical quality*: concerned with the specialist quality of care applied by
  individual providers in their work
- *generic quality*: concerned with the common aspects of quality in the
  way that work is organized and managed, its results and relationships

as applied by whole services or management units (including punctuality, relationships with colleagues and customers and respect for the delivery of the service)
- *systemic quality*: concerned with the quality of a comprehensive and integrated set of services to meet the health needs of a local population, as applied by whole services or management units.

The first two draw upon Donabedian's technical and interpersonal components of care in that they refer to the competence of health care professionals. Generic and systemic quality owe more to industrial models but they are relevant to any organization concerned about communication and cooperation between its component parts, and satisfaction of its internal and external customers.

The total quality management evaluation project drew upon these modes of quality in considering the form of quality assurance that is most appropriate for ensuring high standards of quality for each component. These modes of quality helped us to conceptualize clinical audit at three levels of relevance to clinical care of patients:

- *core clinical audit* refers to assessment of clinical activities directly related to patients that often involve technical activities by therapists
- audit of activity *closely associated* to core clinical practice
- audit of activity *less closely associated* to core clinical practice.

The first level of audit (core clinical audit) addresses technical quality and the other two (closely and less closely associated clinical audit) aspects of generic quality.

In short, changes in emphasis have occurred over time, ranging from absolute to technocratic definitions of quality and thence to quality as a process rather than an attribute of goods or services; a journey rather than a destination. Donabedian's and Maxwell's work contribute substantially to our understanding of health care quality and its assessment. Three modes of quality, technical, generic and systemic are proposed and technical and generic modes are linked to three levels of audit (core clinical, closely associated and less closely associated) to frame our analysis.

We now move to a more specific consideration of the concept of quality assurance.

Quality assurance

As with quality, the term 'quality assurance' is used in several ways. In the context of the NHS it often refers to activities designed to improve the quality of care which lie outside clinical and medical audit (Walshe and Coles 1993). Thus quality assurance refers to the quality of such things as hotel services and the hospital environment and reflects the relatively limited involvement of professionals – particularly doctors – in quality assurance activities. Used in this way quality assurance is often used synonymously with organizational audit.

Walshe and Coles (1993) are critical of this restricted use and suggest that quality assurance is 'more appropriately interpreted as an umbrella term, embracing all aspects of quality measurement and improvement, and including activities such as clinical and medical audit'.

This definition is in line with the use of quality assurance in the broader health care literature in which there is general agreement that quality assurance is a cyclical process with three essential stages: identifying high quality (agreeing expectations and establishing standards or goals), measuring what is happening (auditing performance and function of the organization), and taking action to remedy any discrepancy between the two. Continuous movement through this cycle (or more correctly, a spiral, to imply improvement of quality over time) ensures that quality of care is protected or enhanced.

In later chapters we draw upon the cycle applied to quality assurance as a metaphor, or representation, to assist in our exploration and understanding of clinical audit. We describe and interrogate these cycles and use them to build empirical models which reflect the current state of development of clinical audit in the four professions.

Our reading of the UK literature suggests that the use of quality assurance as a cycle or spiral is increasingly uncommon. Audit and quality assurance seem often to be used interchangeably (in the UK but not in mainland Europe) and the audit cycle has replaced the quality assurance cycle in common parlance.

Quality assurance and quality improvement

Another use of the term 'quality assurance' is to refer to a stage in the development of approaches to maintaining and improving quality, describing an interim period between the eras of quality control and quality improvement.

The period of quality assurance, which began at the end of the Second World War, involved systematic attempts to design out error at every stage of the production process and increased attention to pre-production planning. Most causes of error were apparently located at an earlier stage of the production process than had been thought. So, to improve quality, it was necessary to understand and manage production processes more clearly and effectively. This generated more sophisticated statistical process control methods, the aim of which was to design a process or product that was sufficiently robust to cope with variability in its handling by different machines, workers and consumers. Thus the early statistical processes, that focused on detection of faulty products, were broadened to encompass prevention, but the fundamental approach to policing quality did not change. Individual products were still inspected, often on a sample basis, to see if they met required standards. If not they were re-worked through the production process or scrapped.

As tested by Deming (1991) and Juran (1974) in Japan, quality assurance involved workers more closely than hitherto so that they could contribute to identifying causes of variation and planning changes in work practice to reduce variation. However, it quickly became clear that workers could not easily influence change. For example, problem-solving teams were often intra-departmental and uni-professional and were unable to influence processes that spanned production boundaries or policies and practices that were the province of middle and senior managers.

The response to this was a broadening of quality assurance to encompass all activities within the organization (and later, external suppliers) and vertical extension of quality assurance into the higher reaches of the organization. Quality plans became part of the normal business planning process, quality programmes became increasingly corporate and top-down, and attention was paid to good leadership and producing an organizational framework for quality concerns to flourish. There was also increasing recognition of the need to develop an underlying people-based philosophy of quality (a quality culture) that could support problem solving as a mechanism for continuous quality improvement. Combined with an explicit concern to meet the demands of consumers, many organizations were restructured to make quality everyone's business with the result that quality assurance moved into the era of quality improvement.

The quality improvement literature is dominated by a small number of influential authors, in particular Juran, Deming and Crosby, whose ideas have been picked up and developed by others including a host of management consultancy firms who put forward their own particular model of quality improvement built upon different combinations of empirical observation, research and trial and error. Most authorities emphasize the need for commitment by top managers, worker involvement, systematic efforts to detect and correct errors, continuous effort and sufficient time to establish a culture of continuous improvement.

There are differences between the models. Deming and Juran are statisticians concerned about statistical variation and Deming, in particular, points to the need to understand the nature of variation before making changes to organizational processes. Both place much more emphasis on statistical methods than Crosby, who highlights the need to achieve wide-scale culture change; he emphasizes training and problem-solving tools, and suggests a sequence for implementation. However, Joss *et al.* (1994), referring specifically to total quality management, point out that few conceptual models, Crosby's included, offer advice about how to change the culture of different organizations or take sufficient account of theoretical and conceptual work related to understanding organizations and organizational change.

Over the last two decades government initiatives in installing quality assurance have been mitigated by elements of the quality movement that recognize consumer interests. Pfeffer and Coote (1991) suggest that the concept of quality in the health and welfare services has moved through four chronological stages, each representing a different seat of power:

- *traditional*, representing prestige
- *scientific* or expert, representing normative standards of acceptability
- *managerial*, representing the satisfaction of consumers in competitive markets
- *consumerist*, representing the empowerment and involvement of users.

User interests are still predominantly in the managerial stage, defined and measured as one set of criteria illuminating performance; they are part of a production model in which both professional values and consumer participation are subordinated to measurable and publicly accountable criteria.

In summary, there has been a general progression in both manufacturing industry and commercial services and, more recently in public services, from quality control through quality assurance to quality improvement. Inspection with the purpose of identifying problems and outliers has been gradually replaced with increasingly proactive concern to design quality into the product rather than inspecting it out, together with greater comprehensiveness and attention to creating and maintaining a high quality culture by developing workers and motivating them towards continuous quality improvement. Parallel to this progression has been a movement in the health and welfare services from a traditional prestigious (scientific, normative) approach to quality to the managerial, competitive approach. The consumerist approach, that puts user empowerment high on the agenda, is given lip service but has yet barely managed to maintain a toehold.

Audit

Restricted and broad definitions

'Audit' is a term with precise origins but which has acquired different meanings in relation to health care quality. Derived from *audire*, to hear, audit originally referred to oral accounts of money spent, reflected in dictionary definitions of audit as 'to examine officially', again referring to financial accounts. The origin of the term thus suggests that audit is one stage – the assessment or measurement of quality – within the cycle of quality assurance. This is reflected in much of the health care literature. For example, *Working for Patients* defines medical audit as 'a systematic, critical analysis of the quality of medical care, including the procedures used for diagnosis and treatment, the use of resources, and the resulting outcome for the patient' (Secretaries of State for Health 1989).

Later on in *Working for Patients*, in the section devoted to the health service in Scotland, medical audit is described as 'the systematic process by which doctors continually assess and evaluate their clinical practice, the organisation of services, their managerial function and educational activities.'

These definitions concur with the notion of audit as the measurement necessary to provide doctors with information on quality of care; that is, information that conveys whether improvement in care is required.

Using audit to refer only to the assessment or measurement phase of the audit cycle contrasts with definitions of audit that incorporate both measurement of quality and changing practice when improvement is required. For example, Shaw states that '[m]edical audit, like quality assurance, is a three-part cycle. The first stage is to define expectations, the second is to compare these with observed reality, and the third to bring about appropriate change in clinical practice' (Shaw 1990).

Thus, the broad use of the term takes the concept of audit beyond measurement to incorporate other aspects of the quality assurance cycle.

We therefore distinguish between definitions of audit that are *restricted*, when audit refers to one stage – the measurement of quality – within the cycle of quality assurance; and *broad*, when audit incorporates both measurement of quality and changing practice when improvement is required, and thus goes beyond measurement to incorporate other aspects of the quality assurance cycle.

Both definitions of audit are apparent in government thinking; in some of the professions' literature, restricted and broad uses of the term are used simultaneously. For example, a popular clinical audit manual for speech and language therapists (College of Speech and Language Therapists 1993) defines clinical audit in a restricted way as 'a way of measuring the quality of care provided by a service', but later more broadly as 'quality assurance applied to the clinical activities of any group of health care professionals'.

Clinical audit

Characteristics

Since 1991 medical audit has become firmly established, although research suggests that it is frequently treated as an addition to, rather than an intrinsic part of, medical practice (Kerrison *et al.* 1993). The focus of policy since 1991 has been on involving other professional disciplines, replacing medical audit with the wider concept of clinical audit. This has been the policy adopted by the Department of Health. One interpretation of this approach defines clinical audit as any audit activities that are non-medical. Indeed the emergent phase in medical audit had been closely paralleled by developments within nursing and the therapy professions. Clinical audit was seen as predominantly concerned with service quality; that is, with health care services excluding the medical component (Pollitt 1993b).

The Normand report (Normand *et al.* 1991a, 1991b) chronicled how each of the four professions studied had begun to work on various quality assurance initiatives in the 1980s and 1990s and, through their respective national colleges, had developed guidelines for practice. Ellis and Whittington's (1993) comprehensive study of the development of quality assurance in health care paints a similar picture. The Department of Health certainly recognized that medical and clinical audit were not coterminous. From

1991 central funds had been allocated for audit by the nursing and therapy services, although by 1994 these only totalled £17.7 million, in comparison with the £203 million allocated for medical audit (Department of Health 1993).

But a broader interpretation of clinical audit is that it is essentially multi-professional and, although it may start as a uni-professional process, it aims to involve all health professions in a collective activity:

> We [the Department of Health's Medical Audit Unit] also wondered whether we would succeed in persuading hospital consultants to talk to one another in peer review groups, let alone involve their junior colleagues. Three years later we have developed the culture to the extent that we are able to consider realistically a move in the direction of a much more widespread multi-professional health care audit.
>
> (Marritt 1993)

The Department of Health's use of uni-professional audit to refer to activities in which professions identify their own contribution to patient care (Department of Health 1994a) has not gained currency within the professions and so, for our purposes, clinical audit is regarded as uni- or multi-professional according to whether there is more than one profession involved.

This use of clinical audit may not conform to Department of Health usage, but accords with the spirit of the government's approach. The development of a clinical audit programme that is only multi-professional contradicts the Department of Health's strategy that clinical audit should be developed alongside uni-professional audit.

The Department of Health (1994a) identifies two other key characteristics of successful clinical audit: 'it is focused on the patient'; and 'it develops a culture of continuing evaluation and improvement of clinical effectiveness focusing on patient outcomes'.

Related features of successful clinical audit identified by the Department of Health (1994a) involve:

- it being carried out at health care team level
- making links between health and social services – particularly with respect to vulnerable adults and children living in the community
- encouraging contributions from individual health care professionals
- linking any uni-professional audit activity with overall patient care by the multi-professional team.

The culture of continuing evaluation reflects the current emphasis on quality as continuous improvement. Here, the factors identified as important are appropriateness, timeliness and effectiveness, which refer to whether the correct intervention was instituted at the correct time and in the correct way. Auditing the process is seen as the responsibility of clinical professional groups as part of an overall assessment of multi-professional care.

The focus on outcome casts doubt about the traditional emphasis on inputs and processes in health care (e.g. the number of therapists trained, the number of beds available, whether or not the prescribed procedures are followed). This development follows national and international trends towards outcome measurement. The Department of Health's Clinical Outcome Group is one such initiative.

Features of clinical audit identified by the Department of Health draw upon Donabedian's framework for quality assessment in health care and the current conception of quality as a process of continuous improvement. Our research throws light upon these characteristics of audit as indicators of good practice.

We now move to the ways in which we have found the terms 'audit' and 'clinical audit' to be used by members of the therapy professions.

Definitions of audit used by members of the therapy professions

It will come as no surprise to learn that therapists are no more consistent in their definition of audit as anyone else. Some define clinical audit broadly as a cyclical process concerned with measuring professional activity and incorporating attempts to make quality improvements. Others use a narrower definition in that they see clinical audit as restricted to the measurement of professional activity. This group defines clinical audit as an aspect of quality assurance or as concerned with measurement against predefined standards; they emphasize quantification of activities. A few define the term in an even more restricted sense as simply the collection of information about a service without necessarily any explicit attempt to use this information for measurement purposes. Familiarity with clinical audit is common now although it is not unusual for health care professionals to regard clinical audit as referring to counting and checking things and attending countless meetings.

The distinction between clinical and other forms of audit is not always clear. For some, clinical audit is concerned only with the evaluation of all aspects of the clinical service which impinge upon patient care and treatment. Others distinguish clinical audit, which covers the work of clinicians, from organizational audit, which is to do with other aspects of the service and facilities less closely related to quality of care and treatment.

Some professionals give much greater priority to outcome measurement in clinical audit than others. But there are those who would agree with the view of one therapist who saw clinical audit in process terms, 'audit seems to describe what you do rather than find[ing] out if it [what you do] is effective.'

A distinction is made between clinical audit as either a professional bottom-up activity involving peers and concerned with self-evaluation and professional improvement, or as a top-down management-driven activity concerned with controlling the work of professionals and demonstrating their accountability to purchasers. Professional therapists tend to subscribe to the former view.

It is not unusual for therapy professionals to take a view of audit held by doctors, that audit of the work of doctors is medical audit and audit of the work of other health care professionals is clinical audit. Most therapists, however, use clinical audit to describe their uni-professional audit activities whereas most doctors see clinical audit as a multi-professional activity.

Focus and method of clinical audit

In addition to our distinction between restricted and broad definitions, clinical audit activities can be categorized according to their focus and method. An example of classification by focus, drawn from an information sheet published by the King's Fund (Hunt undated), describes three approaches to audit, all of which are firmly attached to the notion of audit as quality measurement:

- *generic* audit, measuring overall quality in a unit or ward
- *problem-specific* audit, measuring quality related to a clinical topic
- *activity-specific* audit, measuring quality of care provided by a person or group of people.

Methods of audit, or of quality assessment, are diverse. They are often categorized within Donabedian's structure, process and outcome framework (e.g. Hegyvary and Haussman 1976; McMahon 1989) although, as we have seen, Donabedian's categories are not independent and assessment methods are unlikely to fit neatly into any one. For example, some performance indicators reflect the results of health care as outcomes but others address activities and so are process indicators (Fitzpatrick and Dunnell 1992). Patient satisfaction is usually regarded as an outcome of care, but patient complaints and satisfaction surveys often refer to process and structure as well as outcome. As Balogh (1991) points out, the strength of Donabedian's model is that it is iterative; it only makes sense when its features are seen together.

In considering distinctions in focus there has been a shift from *ex post* to *ex ante* forms of evaluation. In *ex post* formats, the objectives for services are set up by professionals, with varying degrees of willingness to listen to the wants and needs of their clients, and evaluation takes place, if at all, retrospectively. It is this that has been the basis of a 'trusting' relationship between the state and professionals. In *ex ante* evaluation, the objectives are pre-set by those who fund and legitimize them, and evaluation takes the form of outcome measures closely related to the predetermined objectives. The first format is consistent with professionally led services and the second with managerially and politically led services.

A sub-set of the *ex ante* form of evaluation is that which depends upon quantitative measures, and particularly performance indicators. These embody assumptions about the desirable outcomes of services which can be geared to objectives. They also assume that a quantitative relationship between the inputs to the service and the outputs of services can be struck.

Thus it becomes possible to determine the degree of value added to what is deemed to be a production process.

Three approaches to auditing health care quality have been identified by Berwick and Knapp (1990):

- *implicit review*, which uses 'experts' who recognize good care (structure, process or outcome) when it occurs
- *explicit review*, which evaluates care against preformulated criteria, often expert-generated, through group discussion or implicit review techniques
- the use of *sentinels*, which defines and investigates unacceptable incidents using implicit or explicit methods. A case review of a patient in a mental health care unit who committed suicide would be an example and the investigation might focus on structure, process and outcome issues.

In implicit review assessors usually work together, often as a peer group, which assumes that the judgement of a group is better than that of an individual. Procedures involve judgements or assessments of quality at varying levels of generality; hence scores may be assigned to records of care or judgements may be made of how well a care system or individual practitioners deal with single clients or groups.

Explicit review can be conducted by non-professional staff who are trained to rate the care, whereas implicit review is likely to be made by health care professionals. Explicit review can be more concise than implicit review, and it may be cheaper if carried out by non-professionals, but it has been criticized for oversimplification and clinical irrelevance (Berwick and Knapp 1990). In general, clinicians favour implicit processes and managers prefer explicit criteria and scoring systems (Berwick and Knapp 1990).

In Chapter 4 we draw upon some of the approaches discussed here to classify clinical audit activities that we have observed. We use the following classification:

- *category* (core clinical activities, closely associated or less closely associated with clinical activities)
- *focus* (structure, process, outcome)
- *nature* (uni- or multi-professional)
- *profession(s)* leading and involved in the audit.

The challenge to health care professionals concerned with quality assessment is to recognize links, in terms of patients' experiences, between the three parts of Donabedian's framework and to identify whether the components of high quality health care have been achieved. Much debate has focused upon the difficulties of establishing causal relationships between process and outcome variables and, more generally, on the complexities of assessing outcomes. For the most part, audit in health care professions other than medicine has focused on structure and process. Medical audit has concentrated on outcomes. Given the current emphasis by the Department of Health on outcome assessment as a means of demonstrating the quality of health care services generally, we now consider it in some detail.

Outcome assessment

In all evaluation systems of health care, economics has played a powerful part. Neo-classical economics provides us with a simple model of health services in which the NHS is regarded as a supplier of health care in response to patient demand. This leads to an economics-based classification for different stages of the health care process:

- inputs to the health care process, including patients, health care staff, buildings and equipment
- intermediate outputs or throughputs: what happens to the patient and care system during treatment
- outputs: the patients as they emerge from treatment
- outcomes of health care: the status of the patient in the long term (e.g. length and quality of life).

This model is helpful conceptually but it oversimplifies the difficulties of outcome assessment. For example, short term outputs (e.g. death of a patient) can also be outcomes (Roberts 1990). For us, Shanks and Frater's (1993) use of outcome simply as a result is preferable because it avoids the need to disentangle outputs from outcomes. Their definition of outcome as a change in health status for which neither the cause nor the nature of the effect is necessarily specified, is useful for most practical purposes. This is a meaningful definition of outcome in the present state of knowledge when we can often measure only the change itself and not its causes. However, a health outcome need not necessarily constitute a change. Maintaining a steady state may be a successful outcome for patients who are frail or who have chronic or progressive disease. Similarly, a reduction in their rate of decline may also constitute a positive outcome.

Measures of health outcome

Health outcome measures can refer to effects at different levels (individuals, local communities or the wider population) and address aspects of health, well-being or quality of life. The following kinds of outcome measure make a useful classification (see Bowling 1991; Long *et al.* 1993):

Quantity of life
Measures commonly used are mortality and avoidable premature mortality. As measures of quality of health, however, they have their limitations in that to be dead might be preferable than to be living in intolerable pain and misery.

Health-related physical, psychological and social aspects of well-being and quality of life
These methods of outcome assessment include measures of:

- functional ability
- pain

- health status
- psychological well-being
- social support
- life satisfaction and morale.

We consider each briefly, giving examples and some indication of their strengths and limitations.

Measures of functional ability   These include direct tests of function (e.g. limb movement, grip strength), observation of a patient's behaviour (e.g. ability to walk, wash) and interviews with the patient/client or carer about the client's independence in activities of living. Often self-report measures are used, such as the Crichton Royal Behaviour Rating Scale (Charlesworth and Wilkin 1982), which assesses the client's functional ability (mobility, feeding, bathing, dressing, continence) and mental disturbance (memory, orientation, communication, cooperation, restlessness).

We should be aware of the limitations of these measures. One drawback is their narrow focus: they cover what service providers consider to be important – mobility, self-care and domestic tasks. They ignore aspects that might be more important to the client, like financial, emotional and social needs.

Measures of pain   Pain is a complex phenomenon to measure and assessment can be hampered by the many misconceptions we all, including professionals, hold about the genuineness of a patient's pain (McCaffery and Beebe 1989). One method of pain assessment that uses a rating scale, a body outline for patients to record the location of their pain and space for comment by patient and carer is the London Hospital Pain Chart (Raiman 1981). This helps the health professional to assess all aspects of the patient's pain, including its nature, its location(s), when it started, its duration, its intensity, its effect on the patient's ability to sleep, to lead an active life, to behave normally, and whether anything makes the pain better.

Measures of health status   These are broader than scales of functional ability or pain and refer to clients' perceptions of their health. Many are self-report scales, such as the Nottingham Health Profile (Hunt *et al.* 1985) and the SF36 (Ware and Sherbourne 1992). Or a simple single item measure is used which asks clients to rate their health as excellent, good, fair or poor. This scale is easy and quick to use and is valid in that it correlates well with morbidity and subsequent mortality (see Bowling 1991 for a review of the literature). The health status scales are more comprehensive but, as with all self-report scales, their scores can be confounded by respondents poor in mental health. That is to say, different scores might emerge for two people, who are considered by clinicians to have a similar health status, because their perceptions of their own health are different.

People who are depressed are likely to rate their health, functional ability and social support as low. Their scores are difficult to interpret because of the problem of disentangling cause and effect.

Measures of psychological well-being   These measures claim to detect aspects of well-being, or 'ill-being', such as anxiety or depression. Examples are the General Health Questionnaire (Goldberg 1978) and the Beck Depression Inventory (Beck *et al.* 1961), both of which have been tested extensively for reliability and validity. For example, the General Health Questionnaire has been validated against independent psychiatric assessment, and is able to detect people who are on the threshold of psychiatric morbidity (see Bowling's review 1991).

Measures of social support   These measures focus on clients' social networks, their self-esteem and whether they feel cared about and loved. A lack of social support is associated with mortality, delayed recovery from illness, poor morale and poor mental health (see Bowling's review 1991). Examples are the Interview Schedule for Social Interaction (Henderson *et al.* 1980) and the Social Network Scale (Stokes 1983). Disadvantages of these scales are their uncertain reliability and validity, which is a problem for all scales that attempt to measure concepts whose definition is elusive and imprecise.

Measures of life satisfaction and morale   The broader and more nebulous the concept, the greater is the difficulty in developing reliable and valid measures. Lack of conceptual clarity is a particular problem for life satisfaction scales because their definition is confounded by related concepts such as happiness, well-being and morale. But some measures are considered reasonably valid, such as the Life Satisfaction Index A (Neugarten *et al.* 1961) and the Affect Balance Scale (Bradburn 1969).

There is no doubt that, as the conceptual definitions underlying these measures become more complex and ambiguous, their validity decreases. But they do achieve some understanding of a person's quality of health, well-being and life and are more useful than simple mortality measures to health professionals in that they can assess the effects of therapeutic interventions over time.

Satisfaction with health care

Monitoring complaints and plaudits and the ubiquitous patient satisfaction surveys are the methods most commonly used to assess satisfaction with health care. Health authorities in England are required to record complaints and respond to them (Department of Health and Social Security 1988). As a measure of satisfaction with care, complaint monitoring is flawed. Only a minority of people complain even when they are critical so that no complaints may not indicate a satisfactory service. Conversely, a high number of complaints does not necessarily convey a bad institution.

Bad institutions might make it so difficult to complain that patients give up the struggle.

The satisfaction survey is a popular method of measuring patients' satisfaction with their care. Early surveys focused on satisfaction with the hotel services (Pollitt 1987) but later studies included satisfaction with technical care, interpersonal care, the environment, accessibility, convenience, cost and so on (e.g. Moores and Thompson 1986). The many limitations to satisfaction scales include their questionable reliability and validity (Bond and Thomas 1992), unwillingness of patients to criticize, particularly when still in hospital, patients' limited knowledge of the services available and their low expectations of the standards that could be achieved (Mangan and Griffiths 1982). For a recent review of patient satisfaction studies, see Batchelor *et al.* (1994).

Processes of health care

Readmission rates, relapses and complications are outcome measures often used to monitor standards of care. They are useful as final outcome measures of the patient's care and treatment as a whole, but they cannot serve as sensitive interim outcome measures when the therapist needs to know how the patient is responding to therapy during the course of treatment as well as at its end.

The problem of validity

Our look at some of the outcome measures available to health professionals shows that there are many to choose from but not all have been established as reliable, valid and responsive (capable of identifying small but important changes). Furthermore, they may not produce meaningful scores that the practitioner can clearly understand and act upon.

In theory the outcomes of any health care service can be assessed but problems can arise in practice. These include difficulties in defining the start and end of treatment, particularly in cases of rehabilitation or continuous treatment for chronic conditions, and difficulties in measuring outcomes of care which have small, but important, effects. The problem here is that outcomes of some interventions are semi-continuous with a large number of small changes gradually leading to other larger changes; so process and outcome variables merge. A practical solution is to refer to inputs or outcomes as intermediate outcomes when their position in a continuing process of care conveys a result. So, for example, a physiotherapist achieves progressively more knee extension with an arthritic patient (intermediate outcomes) which is crucial in achieving the patient's final outcome of being able to walk without pain.

As we have indicated, measuring outcomes can be a methodological minefield. It is helpful to take account of the three general points, emphasized by Long *et al.* (1993), that should be considered in any evaluation of a health care intervention or service:

- a clear definition of the treatment episode
- methods to control for variations in patient characteristics (e.g. severity, age, morbidity) and service variables (e.g. case-mix) and to distinguish the effects of the services to be evaluated from intervening variables from within and outside health services (for example, poverty and housing conditions)
- an adequate data collection period to ensure that all relevant effects appear or a sufficiently large sample is studied.

In Chapter 4 we describe progress made into outcome assessment of patient care and of service provision in the therapy professions.

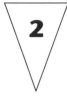

2

Clinical audit and its relationship to other forms of quality assurance and knowledge generation

Tim Packwood and Anémone Kober

The policy context

As we have seen in Chapter 1, clinical audit is one of many forms of quality assurance that has come into prominence as part of a larger movement of thought and action in our public services. Over the last two decades, welfare services in Britain have experienced a degree of questioning and change unparalleled since the 1940s and the creation of the welfare state. This reflects the assertion of new values regarding the desirable role of collective, public services in our society (Bacon and Eltis 1976; Klein and O'Higgins 1985; Gamble 1988; Wilding 1992). This challenge was partly a reaction to perceptions of failure, both general economic failure and the particular inability of welfare services to remedy social ills, and partly a result of the success of the Conservative ideology at the national polls (Flynn 1990).

These challenges have fundamentally altered the ways in which the traditional welfare services, such as education, social services, housing and health, are governed and delivered (Glennerster *et al.* 1991). An important aspect of the new regime has been called 'the rise of the evaluative state' (Neave 1988):

> Government had identified evaluation as a significant component in its strategy to achieve some key objectives: to control public expenditure, to change the culture of the private sector and to shift the boundaries and definition of public and private spheres of activity.
>
> Several changes occurred. New evaluative institutions and practices were installed, based on new assumptions about the knowledge and expertise they required, the values they should endorse and the authority they should carry.

> In particular, government emphasised the technical and instrumental purpose of evaluation by reducing the influence of service-orientated professionals and installing management criteria and expertise.
>
> (Henkel 1991)

In the case of the NHS, the model of governance that emerged post-1945, and was refined in subsequent reorganizations, was that of a weak hierarchical structure of appointed bodies which gave a great deal of discretion, particularly at the local operational level, to professional, and particularly to medical professional, interests (Ham 1992; Klein 1993). Throughout the 1970s and 1980s, increasing attempts were made to make the service more commercially minded. This was accomplished by strengthening service management as a counterweight to professional power, while at the same time emphasizing the importance of commercial principles and processes within public service management (Flynn 1992; Harrison *et al.* 1992). The introduction of general management in 1983, following the Griffiths Inquiry (NHS Management Inquiry 1983), and the launching of the resource management initiative from 1986 onwards (Packwood *et al.* 1991) represent the most significant examples. But these were merely precursors to the far-reaching changes legislated in the NHS and Community Care Act 1990, which separated responsibility for paying for health services from responsibility for their provision, and introduced a regulated internal market into the NHS. The effects were to:

- simplify the government of the service by reducing the former hierarchy (central government, regions, districts, units). Health concerns were now divided below regional level between purchasers (district health authority, commissioning agencies, GP fundholders) and providers (hospitals, community services, primary care services) and those of the latter who gained trust status related directly to central government via management executive outposts, thereby by-passing regional control. In any case, by 1993 regions became a casualty of the government's drive to reduce bureaucracy in the NHS; their reduction in number in 1994 was to be followed by their abolition in 1996. Relationships between purchasers and providers were to be dictated by a quasi-market culture, operationalized through contracts, rather than by a managerial command structure (Le Grand and Bartlett 1993)
- reduce the influence of the professions. They were now, at least partially, susceptible to market forces, having to gain contracts for their work and fulfil the attendant requirements
- strengthen managerial power further. This is perhaps most obvious with reference to the boards of authorities and hospitals, where the senior managers now represent 45 per cent of the membership. But it is also evident through the importance of management in creating and maintaining contracts. Probably of greater long-term significance, the resource management initiative gave service management the potential capability to actively manage clinical work, which is the prime source of demands

for resources on the rest of the service. And the professionals have become increasingly obliged to participate in managing those resources they use, and to account for their use (Packwood *et al.* 1991), reducing further the ethos of collective government in the service. Emphasis has been placed on the rights of individual clients or patients, particularly the right to obtain specific standards of care, as defined by charters or service protocols, and the right to obtain information. Individualism has also been promoted by the encouragement given to individual hospitals and/or community services to become NHS trusts, thereby exercising greater control over their own affairs. Correspondingly, the influence of bodies that might express collective values, such as community health councils (tenuous at best) and local authorities, has been diminished.

It is against this setting that the health service has experienced a wide range of quality initiatives over the years. Largely in the *ex post* mode, described in Chapter 1, are the Health Advisory Service, dating from 1969 and the National Development Team for People with a Mental Handicap, which was created in 1976 (Henkel *et al.* 1989). The more recently stressed *ex ante* mode (see Chapter 1) is represented by the National Audit Office which, since 1983, has been concerned that health service expenditure is both in accordance with the 'will of Parliament' and is securing value for money (Harrison 1992).

The Audit Commission extended its field of operations to include the health service as part of the 1989 health and community care reforms. The best-known recent initiatives are those in medical audit. As we discuss later, these have been primarily conceived as an educational device in which medical staff, by sharing discussion of the outcomes of treatment, learn from each other. But there is evidence that the *ex post* and *ex ante* debate continues, in that managers are also concerned that medical audit should provide data upon which they can make judgements about the efficacy of services and use of resources. They need to know what standards and criteria are being adopted beforehand so that they can judge cost effectiveness.

A further significant initiative, as we have mentioned in Chapter 1, has been the introduction of total quality management in the NHS. This involved the funding of 17 projects, some of which divided into more than one site later on, and the systematic evaluation of their success. Total quality management admits to several and conflicting definitions; a recent study indicates the commonalities:

There is no single or succinct definition of total quality management. The principal authors tend to define total quality management according to their own ideas of its desired outputs. Taken together, the different versions add up to an integrated, corporately-led programme of organisational change designed to engender and sustain a culture of continuous improvement based on customer-oriented definitions of quality. The main features include:

- integrated corporate planning both for operations and for quality;
- organisational structures for quality improvement to ensure:
  accountability for quality improvement; and
  supporting staff for quality improvement;
- staff empowerment to create a quality-aware and motivated staff
  skilled in process improvement;
- models and methods for systematic measurement and evaluation;
- movement towards a common definition of quality;
- customer-oriented definitions of quality.

(Joss *et al.* 1994)

Other initiatives have been: resource management, standards setting in nursing and the therapy professions, the spread of accreditation by BS5750, and the King's Fund organizational audit scheme, which was seen as acting as a catalyst for quality in those institutions where it was applied. Consumerism, too, has become a stronger influence in the NHS over the last quarter-century. This has not been so much a product of public representation and participation, as of managerial and political initiatives. Examples would include the recommendations of the Griffiths Report (NHS Management Inquiry 1983) and latterly the powerful changes introduced by purchasers and the requirements of the Patient's Charter. These last have required regions, districts and units to make regular returns to the Department of Health on the extent to which certain national objectives, such as reduction of waiting lists, have been achieved.

Quality requirements are now routinely included in the contracts being made by purchasers of services from trusts and other health units. The observation of our colleague team which has been concerned with evaluating the total quality management pilot experiment (Joss *et al.* 1994; Joss and Kogan 1995) is that there is a mass of quality work being undertaken throughout the health service, some of it highly innovatory and determined. But their study also identified a lack of cohesion between initiatives made from the centre or locally, a tendency for initiatives to start at the professional and operational base but not always to be mandated by management, and uncertainty about the technical bases of quality assurance, particularly on such issues as outcome measurement. Nor have the links between attempts to define and measure quality and the creation of appropriate organizational structure been strong enough.

In spite of these major changes important continuities also remain. From its genesis the NHS has had to stretch every pound; demand has always exceeded supply (Klein 1993). The creation of an internal market does not remedy the resource problem; it rather places the responsibility for allocation of available services with a different set of actors, with the purchasers rather than with the Department of Health. But there seems little evidence that the centre actually wishes to relinquish its responsibility. Far from reducing hierarchical and bureaucratic influences, the recent changes can be interpreted as making them more effective, removing, in the familiar tradition of organizational consultancy, unnecessary levels of management and improving the capacity to manage what remains. Now that the centre presides over two short hierarchies of purchaser and provider services, rather than one long multipurpose hierarchy, its potential for exercising strategic management appears to have vastly increased. The belated recognition that the centre has a management task to perform, as evident in the creation of the Management Executive and its separation (geographical as well as functional and cultural) from the traditional policy advisory task, is surely crucial in this respect.

A further continuity can be seen in terms of policy. Community care has been a priority, if somewhat implicit and rhetorical (Ham 1992), for over two decades. And the motivations – the increasing numbers of chronically ill, consumer choice, new fashions in treatment and care, development of medical technology and care – are all as important today as ever (Walker 1989). Indeed it is possible that the pressures of the internal market for cost-effective use of specialized facilities will increase the incentive to treat chronically ill people outside hospitals.

The emergence of audit

The development of audit in the NHS illustrates the interplay of all the themes and tensions displayed above. It emerged in the 1970s and 1980s as a predominantly professional activity and as a predominantly medical professional activity. It was promoted by a number of enthusiasts and gradually gained acceptance and support from the medical establishment (Kerrison *et al.* 1993). Audit in this 'emergent phase' could be characterized as fragmented, professionally encapsulated and formative in its intent; a way of improving individual practice through collective knowledge. Distinctions between audit and research or audit and professional educational devices, such as 'grand ward rounds', were unclear.

But during this emergent phase audit was also being viewed from a rather different standpoint. Evidence was accumulating of wide variations in medical practice, and pressures on health resources were intensifying as the economy moved into recession (Pollitt 1993a). Audit could provide a mechanism by which doctors would be persuaded to consider the efficiency and effectiveness of their actions, and whether they were securing value for money. In his report, which had led to the strengthening of management in the NHS, Griffiths had urged the case for doctors evaluating their practice as a means of assessing effectiveness and public accountability (NHS Management Inquiry 1983). Professionals' engagement in audit was a key component of the resource management initiative that followed; for, if professionals were to exercise greater responsibility for the management of their own activities, it had to be on the basis of knowing what they were doing and with what effects. The new computer systems required to provide the activity data for resource management could also serve as a data bank for audit (Packwood *et al.* 1991). In 1988 the Social

Services Select Committee advocated the importance of assessing clinical performance and made a direct connection between the evidence of medical audit and improvement in the use of resources (Social Services Committee 1988; Flynn 1992).

This vision of audit is rather more managerial than the earlier versions, more summative in its nature, and concerned with resource use as a means of securing value for money. And it was this latter vision that appeared dominant in *Working for Patients* setting out the proposed reforms (Secretaries of State for Health 1989) and in the immediate explanations that followed on its publication (NHS Review Working Paper 1989). As we have noted in Chapter 1, medical audit, for significantly the concern was explicitly only with doctors, was defined as 'a systematic critical analysis of the quality of medical care, including the procedures used for diagnosis and treatment, the use of resources, and the resulting outcome for the patient' (Secretaries of State for Health 1989).

Although it was also conceded that medical audit is 'essentially a professional matter' it was made clear that all doctors were required to participate and that, at the local operational levels of the service at least, medical audit was a managerial concern. District management was responsible for ensuring that medical audit took place. Managers had a right to be informed of the results of audit and, if they felt that their concerns were not being met by the existing arrangements, they could initiate independent audits. A hierarchical system of audit committees, stretching from unit to region, and including management representation, was subsequently created to allocate audit monies and supervise the process (Department of Health 1991c; Packwood *et al.* 1992a).

But somewhere between 1989 and 1991 the harder view of the purpose of audit became blunted. Explanations may be sought in the change of personalities at the helm of government in the Department of Health, in the approach of a general election or in the fact that the medical profession had largely accepted the principle of audit and was not at such odds with the government over this, as over other aspects of the reforms. In any event, the managerial emphasis became muted, and greater stress was placed on audit as a 'matter for the medical profession' and as 'primarily an educational activity' (Department of Health 1991c).

Although the logic of audit was argued as a bottom-up activity, performed locally by clinicians grouped according to their specialist interests, there was always a top-down element. The national professional bodies were encouraged by government to play a role in supporting and stimulating local audit (Kerrison *et al.* 1994). Specialist groups created under the auspices of, or working in association with, the Royal Colleges, were devoting effort to the formulation of protocols and guidelines. These had potential for the management of clinical activities and it could be speculated that the possibility of strong professional control of audit was a factor in causing the government to 'soft pedal' on imposing managerial control.

Monies for medical audit were earmarked and distributed either to the regions for local allocation, or to the national professional bodies. And a new disciplinary group, medical audit support staff, were called into existence to assist the doctors with the mechanics of the process.

From 1991 funds had been allocated for audit by the nursing and therapy services although, as noted in Chapter 1, by 1994 these only totalled £17.7 million, in comparison with the £203 million allocated for medical audit (Department of Health 1993). Such a move accepted the principle that the provision of care in the NHS was a multi-professional activity, and that to audit each profession's contribution separately might be wasteful and counterproductive. Contracts were increasingly framed in terms of services to patients, not services provided by individual professions. And staff were increasingly organized on the basis of multi-professional groupings (directorates, departments, care groups) providing patient services (surgery, orthopaedics), services for those with learning disabilities or services in support (pathology) (Packwood *et al.* 1992b). Hence the setting up of the Clinical Outcomes Group referred to in Chapter 1.

The Department's vision of the development of clinical audit is stated as 'largely multi-professional and part of a wider quality management programme that spans all aspects of care in hospitals and in the community' (Department of Health 1993).

The professional and managerial interpretations of audit appear to be reaching symbiosis, for although 'the managerial contribution to clinical audit will be enhanced', it is also accepted that 'clinical audit must remain clinically led and educationally based', and that 'the practice of audit remains a professional activity' (Department of Health 1993).

The adjustment from uni-professional to multi-professional audit received similarly balanced treatment: '[t]he move to multi-professional working should take place at a pace which participants at local level find consistent with the development of uni-professional standards and values' (Department of Health 1993).

But this may understate the difficulties that arise in working together. Not only do the relative statuses of the various professions in the health service differ but medical practitioners have placed emphasis on outcome analysis, whereas other health professions, at least thus far, have emphasized process analysis. By 1994, however, the Department of Health was defining clinical audit as a generic activity which was to encompass both uni- and multi-professional audits (Department of Health 1994a).

The new financial arrangements for clinical audit from 1994 marked a considerable change. First, monies were to be allocated by the management executive to regions, and by regions to purchasers, districts or commissioning agencies, on the same basis as other revenue allocations, namely the resident population to be served. Second, it was suggested that purchasers negotiate contracts for clinical audit from the providers by grouping together and getting one of their numbers to act as 'lead purchaser' and place a 'block contract' with the provider for clinical audit activities.

This would enable purchasers to agree, and require, that specific audit activities be undertaken and to review the results achieved. However, the proposed arrangements also attempted a further balance, in so far as the contract should reflect both purchasers' and providers' priorities. It was claimed that this arrangement 'allows audit to address more adequately questions of health care needs and health care effectiveness and to become fully integrated in the mainstream business of provider units/trusts/primary care and health purchasing authorities' (Department of Health 1994b).

Accompanying advice from the Department of Health raises a suspicion that, in the course of its short history as a government policy, audit has combined so many purposes as to take on the character of a universal panacea (Department of Health 1994a). Health professionals should take the lead on audit, but it should also examine cost effectiveness and value for money at the clinical team level as part of the business planning function. It should contribute to professional education, to professional integration, should involve general managers and develop the role of the purchaser, look across the primary/secondary care interface and should include an input from patients and carers.

Strong arguments can be advanced for using audit for any of the above purposes; the doubt must be as to how far a relatively small working process can hope to satisfy so many aspirations.

As far as the four therapy professions, whose experience of audit forms the subject of this book, are concerned, all have inevitably been affected by the enormous changes in the NHS as a working environment since 1989. All, too, have been affected by the associated alterations in status and power vis-á-vis other interests. In particular:

- the therapy professions have had to adjust to the move towards general, and away from functional, management. Formerly the therapy professions worked in a hierarchy headed at the apex by a manager from their own discipline. This senior manager might, therefore, be expected to assert and maintain the particular values of the profession concerned. Now the apex, and perhaps the level below the apex, will be occupied by a general manager drawn from any NHS, or non-NHS, discipline. And at lower levels of the hierarchy, members of the profession may find their accountability divided: operationally accountable to a local general manager, professionally accountable to a senior member of their own discipline (Øvretveit 1992; Packwood et al. 1992b)
- in association with the above changes, management controls over professional activity have increased, both in number and strength. Contracts and their various requirements shape and limit professional freedoms. Trusts are beginning to take advantage of their own freedoms in the NHS structure to fashion their own working conditions, thereby restricting the former freedoms of some of their employees. And managerial reactions and local initiatives in respect of the new emphasis on quality and customer satisfaction mean that professionals find themselves

part of quality assurance structures that impose further, and sometimes conflicting, managerial control (Joss *et al.* 1994)

- professional workers, and particularly those occupying senior positions, are having to devote more time to management activities; marketing their services, defining, costing, recording and controlling service activities, managing a budget and engaging in audit and other forms of quality assurance. All of these demands, although legitimate, may be seen as reducing the time available for patient care
- the internal market and its associated changes have also meant some devolution of authority to the various therapy professions to develop services according to their own perceptions of need and demand. They have become less bound by bureaucratic procedures and service traditions.

But, as we discovered in our research, the greatest contextual influence experienced by members of the four therapy professions is that of having to live with continual change. Change can provide a challenge and stimulation, and certainly staff in the therapy professions have succeeded in making the new arrangements work and in achieving improvements in service performance. But this all carries a cost; change can also invoke a threat and uncertainty. Many of our respondents felt that change had been continuous since 1989, as units experienced fusion and fission and services were reshaped in different combinations. Professional practitioners were having to learn to work in new ways, and were having to forge relationships with new groupings and interests in the local environment. All of this takes time and energy and was seen, by some, as self-defeating in that the pressure of adjusting to the next demand detracts from the ability to master the processes concerned with the last requirement. Clinical audit depends upon the creation and maintenance of a structured cyclical process, and this lack of stability adds considerably to the complexity of audit activities.

Given this background, what are now the connections between clinical audit, quality assurance and other forms of audit and what are the links between research and audit?

Connections between clinical audit and quality assurance

In particular, we need to ask whether clinical audit and other forms of audit connect, and if so, how do they connect. The possibilities are:

- merger or incorporation of clinical audit into medical audit
- loose connections between various forms of audit
- clinical audit as 'free-floating', with no real connections
- incorporation of all forms of audit into clinical audit.

We also need to ask at what level do they connect, and is the form of connection

- uni-professional?
- multi-professional?
- organizational?

What implications do these connections – or lack of them – have for the status and profile of clinical audit? Is there a high or a low level of integration of clinical audit within the wider quality assurance framework? How do audit and research overlap, interact and complement each other? And how does audit contribute to knowledge generation? We shall develop this theme at the end of the chapter.

We have explained how clinical and medical audit form part of a wide range of quality assurance initiatives launched by the Department of Health in recent years. But how can we define the differences between clinical and medical audit and the other forms of quality assurance? They are distinguishable from the others inasmuch as the two forms of audit are concerned to demonstrate efficacy in different patterns of clinical care. Other forms of quality assurance may take up the audit of clinical care as an important ingredient in the pursuit of other forms of quality, but they do not aim to work at the clinical heart of health processes in the same way as do the audit procedures.

Total quality management encompasses the *generic* and *systemic* elements of quality assurance (Joss *et al.* 1994). As noted in Chapter 1, by generic we mean those aspects of quality which should apply to all groups working within the health service, for example, attitudes towards patients and modes of working with other professionals and other groups within a health service unit. Systemic aspects of quality concern the ability of a whole unit or trust to work towards shared objectives, to make an efficient distribution of resources, and to establish and maintain appropriate systems for achieving objectives.

Clinical and medical audit are concerned primarily, but not necessarily exclusively, with the clinical processes and outcomes of patient care; in other words, largely with the technical mode of quality assurance, also with interpersonal interaction in the case of clinical procedures.

This may involve, however, both generic and systemic aspects of care. How can this be? The results of a clinical audit could legitimately include concern with the contexts in which clinical care takes place. It might lead to questioning of how long patients wait for treatment. It might analyse how far customers' definitions of need are incorporated into the audit process, or the extent to which a particular professional group shares definitions of quality made for the whole organization. It might lead to questioning about the reduction in inter-professional barriers, as well as the reduction in errors and waste. It might also be concerned with the provision of enhanced management information.

These are not the primary focus of clinical audit, but clinical audit might trigger them off. All of these are deemed to be the primary foci of total quality management, but form at least contextual concerns within which clinical care is pursued and evaluated.

By the same token, such quality assurance initiatives as the Patient's Charter form part of second- or third-order concerns of clinical audit. The Patient's Charter has been primarily concerned with operational procedures which ensure that patients do not wait unduly for treatment. It might be concerned with reducing inter-professional barriers and, through its concern with analysing processes affecting patients, might also concern itself indirectly with the reduction of error and waste.

The *resource management initiative* has presumptions of indirect links to patients' care but is not in any sense concerned with the technical evaluation of that care. It could be assumed, however, that clinical audit, in determining the efficacy of care, would ultimately contribute towards evaluating the effective use of resources, which is part of the resource management process.

Organizational audit, as practised in the King's Fund project, has brought audit in general to the attention of many practitioners and is beginning to be practised in an increasing number of sites. It is, however, primarily concerned with generic and systemic issues.

A further indirect form of quality assurance is that associated with *compulsory competitive tendering* and the *making of contracts*. In these, clinical and medical audit would offer the initial criteria by which tendering and contracting would be judged. Purchasers are required to incorporate the results of audit in their thinking about tendering and contracting.

We can thus discern a clearly defined role for clinical audit in this array of quality assurance devices. Its function is primarily the improvement of clinical practice. But the data resulting from audit might form some of the criteria by which quality assurance of many different kinds is judged to be effective. At the same time, there is a clear logical line between care of patients and the larger organizational and social contexts within which health professionals work. We shall return to the operational significance of these links when we examine care and audit cycles and other sequences in Chapter 3.

Organizational structures for a quality assurance framework

Generally, audit activities tend to be one-off and isolated events. Neither, in most sites, is there an overall quality assurance framework. When audit activities operate together across working units they are usually uni-professional.

Not all general or professional managers, in fact, feel that an overall, unit-wide quality framework is the best option. In sites, for example, with no quality department the aim could be for quality to become an integral part of each service, rather than a separately stimulated activity. Each service would have its own business plan that would outline its quality objectives. But most senior managers would sponsor the need to integrate clinical audit, medical audit and other forms of quality assurance, even if this integration was in fact still at the planning stage.

Practice varies. In one site, the new chief executive wanted to create a general quality assurance system, a large part of which would be multi-professional clinical audit. Audit would be connected to generic and systemic concerns, and led as much by the clinicians as the managers. In another site, senior managers felt that it was for them to develop a more integrated approach to clinical audit across the trust on the grounds that there were enormous hidden costs to uncoordinated audit activities. Even if there were professional resistances to the breaking down of barriers between medical and other types of clinical audit, it was felt that management's hand would be strengthened by the fact that from April 1994 audit monies would no longer be ring-fenced as before (NHS Management Executive 1993; Department of Health 1994b).

In yet another site, there was an overall programme for organizational development in the trust. The plan was to set up ten frameworks, one of which would be quality, with values and mission statements. At the time of fieldwork, however, the approach to quality was patchy.

Obviously, the approach to clinical audit and its integration with other forms of quality assurance varies according to the role perceived by general managers and leading professionals respectively.

Links with medical audit

Medical audit has at present a much higher profile than clinical audit among provider unit general managers and purchasers, and is better integrated in the overall structure of the unit. Many units have medical audit committees. In some sites, senior managers and professionals sit on these committees, thus giving management access to audit data. In others, medical audit committees meet regularly and their members include chief executives, head clinicians in each specialty, chairmen and the full-time staff who run audit. We have found examples of good liaison between management and doctors, who accept that management had a need to have access to audit data.

The higher profile of medical audit in the sites could be due to the following reasons:

- the more advanced stage of medical audit. It was developed earlier and was allocated generous finances and support facilities
- a structure being in place, often with committees at unit level because medical audit has become virtually prescribed practice
- the greater status of the medical profession and its motivation to maintain control of medical audit
- the relatively small number of therapists in the health service.

Generally, there are few strong links between medical audit and clinical audit. This may be because medical audit has primarily been used as a developmental and educational tool internal to the profession (Packwood 1991) rather than for purposes of public accountability.

Links between medical and clinical audit depend on many structural and organizational factors. Where a strong medical culture exists, there are usually weak links between medical and clinical audit, with clinical audit having lower status and less importance in the organization. Therapists, too, may be aware of the greater resources available for medical audit and this could create resentment.

Conversely, where the medical audit culture is less dominant, stronger connections may develop between medical and clinical audit. Some clusters of specialties (psychiatry, rehabilitation, learning disabilities) seem to promote much closer team working, which is conducive to the development of multi-professional audit.

In our study, doctors, particularly those working closely with members of other professions in the delivery of care (e.g. psychiatrists, geriatricians), welcomed a move to multi-professional clinical audit. Other doctors, for example surgeons, were more resistant. This may have to do with the fact that in some specialties there is a clear differentiation of task between different professions.

Possible ways of making the link can be found. The chair of the medical audit committee could sit on both the trust audit committee and the Patient's Charter committee. Medical audit would then become more closely integrated with other quality work and clinical audit. We have encountered plans to create a clinical audit committee at trust board level that would include the chief executive and some senior general managers, representatives from the professions (nursing, medicine, the therapies) and the quality department. The aims of the committee would be to coordinate audit projects, determine priorities and allocate funding. Elsewhere, in a community mental health unit, medical audit had started to move into multi-professional clinical audit. The development of medical audit in this unit had been slow and multi-professional clinical audit encapsulated medical audit.

Clinical audit has tended to be treated as essentially a 'free-floating', uni-professional activity, relatively low in status compared to medical audit. It has been rather piecemeal, the work of individual professions, and with few connections between them. Most sites do not have an organizational structure for clinical audit nor an overview of it. In many sites, too, there is no systematic consideration of clinical audit reports by the trust board.

Links with nursing audit

Nursing audit has been primarily either management controlled using generic audit tools, or has involved bottom-up standards setting using, for example, the RCN's Dynamic Standards Setting System (Royal College of Nursing Standards of Care Project 1989). There is some movement by nurses now to progress beyond standards setting exercises into quality assessment projects that focus on effectiveness of their care on patient outcome using measurement. Mostly nursing audit is under the control of its own professional management. It essentially involves standards setting by the nurses and auditing these standards.

We have found attempts to integrate nursing audit with therapy audit. This had been resisted by some therapists at one region, who wanted to keep the regional audit coordinator's post separate from nursing concerns and develop clinical audit in the therapy professions independently from nursing audit.

On the whole, there are no formal links between clinical audit by the therapists and nursing audit, although nurses and therapists worked together in most of the multi-professional audit projects we investigated.

Links with quality assurance departments

Most sites have not developed links between clinical audit and quality assurance departments and their staff at provider unit level. Audit and quality facilitators, where they exist, often have trust-wide functions to develop a quality framework and culture. They work with professionals and liaise with purchasers and are usually accountable to a general manager.

Often, however, quality facilitators and directors have little influence, or even knowledge, of existing clinical audit activities in the four professions. This is not surprising considering the low level of integration of clinical audit in the wider organization. In one site, however, the quality facilitator was a therapist who had knowledge of most audit projects in the therapy professions.

Quality assurance departments have more links with medical audit. In several sites, the director of nursing and quality (or a similar post holder) was a member of the medical audit committee. This ensures some linkage between the quality assurance department and medical audit. The ability of these quality staff to influence medical audit is, however, limited.

It seems that several factors inhibit the development of a framework that will integrate clinical audit and other forms of audit:

- the lack of clear mechanisms
- the piecemeal, underdeveloped, nature of much clinical audit
- some rivalry between professions
- the lack of adequate information systems, which prevents the integration of outcome measures into broader systemic concerns.

Another inhibitor is the frequent lack of a common view on audit between general managers and professionals, and between professionals: 'there isn't really a consensus as regards audit. Managers have a different definition of audit from health professionals. Nursing defines audit as a top-down prescribed strategy whereas doctors have a more democratic approach and try to set standards together. Therapists are somewhere in between' (consultant geriatrician).

These various issues need to be addressed for a multi-professional clinical audit framework to develop. In the sites as we saw them, however, clinical audit had developed as an essentially non-medical audit activity.

Connections with purchasers

Links between purchasers and providers have grown slowly and until now purchasers have played a minimal role in setting the clinical audit agenda. With the change in the allocation of clinical audit funds, however, purchasers will become increasingly involved in selecting topics, promoting development and monitoring results of clinical audit. Hence it is important to analyse further existing and potential connections between purchasers and providers.

The purchasers have the following range of functions: prescribing standards for contracts, monitoring, facilitating, needs assessment and epidemiology and providing public knowledge about health. In our view, clinical audit could be better exploited in the performance of these tasks. Following Rein (1983), we can call clinical audit 'hot' knowledge. The use of 'hot' knowledge for purchasers might be related to contracts or be used as feedback information for needs assessment. These two tasks are considered in some detail below.

Contracting

If, in our study, there were few links between purchasers and providers, the negotiation and setting of contracts was often emphasized as the way through which quality could be specified and assured. Contracting is one of the principal means by which links between purchasers and providers can be developed.

Quality standards set in contracts have been on the whole unsophisticated and more concerned with quantity and waiting lists than quality of the service. Unit quality standards need to be more closely integrated into the terms of contracts. In the words of a chief executive: 'the quality initiatives in place at the moment are not relating closely enough to the contracts'.

There may also be a gap between the level of the quality standards set in the contracts and the ability to translate these into practice at provider level. On the whole, connection and negotiation between providers and purchasers has not been achieved.

Purchasers are also felt to lack knowledge but professionals have been noted as informing and educating purchasers about what clinical criteria to include in the contracts.

Needs assessment

Clinical audit data can feed back to needs assessment and inform allocations. Needs assessment can be the link as far as knowledge generation between purchasers and providers is concerned.

Purchasers have a formal responsibility to define health and health care needs in the total population. These are global needs which relate to systemic modes of quality assurance (epidemiology). Specific needs, on the other hand, can be defined by professionals and are part of technical and generic modes of quality assurance. However, patient or client needs do not necessarily coincide with professionally defined needs (Bradshaw 1972; Packwood and Whitaker 1988; Davies and Kober 1991).

Purchasers often do not have the systems and knowledge in place to determine specific clinical needs. They cannot easily assess needs without the help of the professionals who are in contact with the patients. Although professionals have no formal responsibility to define population needs, they may contribute to knowledge generation through clinical audit and feed back the information to purchasers. From the professionals' point of view, the process would move from assessing patient needs to setting goals, to intervention, to measurement and to reassessment in order to find out if needs have been met.

There is now a commercial rift between purchasers and providers, increased by the fact that provision of information could be seen as weakening the providers' position in the market. There is a need for better channels of communication between providers and purchasers.

There is also a need for better communication between providers, purchasers and patients, so that purchasers and providers become informed about patient-defined needs. Some client groups may convert into interest groups presenting demands on providers and purchasers for particular forms of audit. There was some embryonic evidence of this in one site.

Thus, links between providers and purchasers are still at a relatively undeveloped stage. However, contracting and needs assessment constitute potentially important areas of cooperation between providers, purchasers and patients.

Connecting clinical audit to the wider organizational framework

There are several levels of connection possible and desirable between clinical audit and the wider organizational framework. Clinical audit can occur within a service and connect the professionals, the service manager and, increasingly, the patients. At a broader level, clinical audit can connect several services and link in with general management, purchasing units and non-NHS organizations (e.g. social services, education).

Batstone (1994) developed a model showing the different levels of maturity of medical audit. On the same lines, it is possible to distinguish several levels in the development of clinical audit, although the different levels do not necessarily correspond to a chronological history of clinical audit, or a move from uni- to multi-professional audit. Some of the main levels of connections, their corresponding modes of quality assurance and examples of prerequisites are presented in Table 2.1.

Table 2.1 Connections of clinical audit (for uni- or multi-professional clinical audit)

Essential connections	Organizational level	Mode of quality assurance	Examples of prerequisites
1 Connecting the clinical audit cycle with the patient care and standards setting cycles	• intra-service • possibly supra-organizational (e.g. national standards set by professional bodies)	• technical • generic	• clinical knowledge base of professionals • knowledge on audit and quality issues/methods • authority of the professional service manager/team leader to effect change within the service
2 Connecting the four cycles (clinical audit, patient care, standard-setting, change cycles)	• essentially intra-service	• technical • generic • systemic	• connections between the professional service manager/team leader and general management • clear lines of accountability for audit
3 Connecting clinical audit with other forms of audit and quality assurance	• intra-service and/or inter-service	• technical • generic • systemic	• unit-wide quality/audit committee ensuring connections between the different groups (quality assurance staff, providers, professional service managers, general managers) • unit-wide data system • clear lines of accountability for audit
4 Connecting clinical audit with purchasers	• intra-service and/or inter-service	• technical • generic • systemic	• unit-wide quality/audit committee, including purchasers • possibly direct connections between purchasers and providers • unit-wide data system • clear lines of accountability for audit
5 Connecting clinical audit with non-health service groups/organizations	• inter-service	• technical • generic • systemic	• unit-wide quality/audit committee, including representatives from consumers and non-NHS providers and purchasers • clear lines of accountability for audit • cross-organizational data system

Clinical audit and knowledge generation

Clinical audit produces data and generates knowledge which are of interest to a variety of stake-holders: health professionals, patients, general managers and purchasers, but also researchers and education professionals. Three main aspects of knowledge and knowledge generation concern us here: the links between audit and research, audit and education, and the dissemination of audit knowledge.

Clinical audit and research

Relatively few respondents commented on the links between audit and research. Of those who did, many felt that audit and research addressed different topics, had different purposes and used different methods: 'research for me is doing a formal project using an unbiased methodology and producing unbiased results. Research needs to be demonstrated – audit is looking at your own service and it [audit] might not be structured, you might not have a random sample' (senior physiotherapist).

One respondent felt that audit was more difficult than research, as it addresses topics in a 'real life' situation: '[with audit] the challenge is developing effective and useful systems of looking at what one is doing as an ongoing part of a real clinical situation . . . the difficulty is actually designing something that can be done as part of work' (head of psychology rehabilitation).

Rather than directly compare clinical audit with research, we have attempted to summarize some of the main characteristics of a clinical audit in Table 2.2.

Research is often deductive and concerned with critical testing. Control groups and validated measures are more likely to be used in research than audit. Audit is often concerned with small-scale problems requiring local solutions. The scope of research is likely to be different and to reach a wider national and international audience through publication of results in academic journals.

Research can provide answers in areas that audit could not tackle and challenges the efficacy of a particular therapy. It raises questions about purposes (and means of achieving them). Audit evaluates what exists and takes purposes for granted. It ascertains whether the inputs and processes achieve the outcome desired.

Audit and research can feed into each other. Audit can give rise to research questions; if the outcomes of audit are not what is intended, research can ask why: 'audit has probably led me to see the way for more research' (district speech and language therapist).

We have encountered at least two audit projects described as audit *and* research. The first one was concerned with the extent to which occupational therapy contributed to keep elderly people in the community. The other one, also in occupational therapy, was just starting and was concerned with outcomes in an elderly care unit.

Table 2.2 The main characteristics of clinical audit

1 Topics	• relevant to the local situation • relevant to career/patient/professional
2 Purpose	• evaluation • monitoring • better patient care • effective use of resources • knowledge (as a complement to research and in its own right, pointing to new areas for research)
3 Time-scale	• short (need for quick results and feedback)
4 Methodology	• measurement against implicit or explicit standards • opportunistic: makes use of existing data (e.g. patients' notes, statistical returns, waiting lists, computerized databases etc.) • not necessarily controlled or validated (e.g. non-representative questionnaire surveys etc.)
5 Feedback and dissemination	• local (professionals, managers in the provider unit, purchasers, region) • national (conferences, professional bodies)
6 Mechanisms of feedback, dissemination	• internal reports (service level, provider unit level, purchaser level, regional level) • audit meetings at service/unit level • results presented at national or regional audit conferences • results of some (but far from all) audit projects are published
7 Impact	• mainly local (within the unit)

Clinical audit and education

Clinical audit is, among other things, a professional development activity. Some respondents felt that clinical audit had highlighted their education needs in relation to audit methods and data analysis. Some felt that attending courses on audit would improve their knowledge of audit and also enhance professional performance. It was suggested that if one person in a team attended such a course, he or she could then disseminate this knowledge to colleagues.

By generating new knowledge, clinical audit could also contribute to post- and undergraduate curricula in the health care professions. In the words of one respondent: 'clinical audit can help to identify areas where there are shortfalls in knowledge and where the education provided to professionals does not match service requirements . . . There is a need to adapt education to the changing nature of the elderly population' (general manager, elderly/physically disabled services).

Two-directional links could be established with education professionals. Health professionals would provide knowledge on existing clinical needs and on change occurring in this area. Education providers could use this knowledge to adapt curricula to new requirements, whilst providing health professionals with advice on research methods.

This chapter has focused on the connections of clinical audit with other forms of quality assurance and on issues related to knowledge generation and dissemination. Chapter 3 examines the value of the notion of a cycle to represent clinical audit.

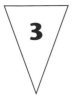

3 Making a start on clinical audit: cycles and spirals

Ian Norman

In creating an audit procedure we need a framework that will help practitioners and managers to envisage the sequence of clinical audit and the interconnections between its stages. The conventional way of presenting audit is as a cycle (e.g. Shaw 1990; Crombie and Davies 1993) in which current practice is compared against a standard. If care is found to be less than satisfactory, attempts are made to introduce change to improve its quality. This metaphor of the cycle is often applied to clinical audit (the clinical audit cycle) and is elaborated and extended here to care of clients and their families (patient care cycle), to standards setting (the standards setting cycle) and to change (the change cycle).

In this chapter we describe the cycles and interrogate them for their feasibility and coherence. We developed a process of analysis which can be found in the annex to Chapter 5. Our final conclusions and recommendations from this analysis are presented in Chapter 7.

The cycles described

Clinical audit cycle

Taking the broader definition of audit (see Chapter 1), we have conceived audit as a cyclical process comprising six stages (Figure 3.1):

- identifying a problem or issue
- establishing standards and goals
- assessing or measuring what is happening (auditing performance and function of the organization) to determine if standards are met
- identifying the change needed

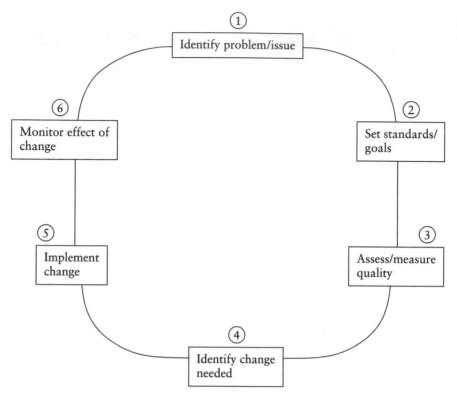

Figure 3.1   The clinical audit cycle (CAC)

- implementing change
- monitoring its effects.

Continuous movement through this cycle ensures that quality of care is protected or enhanced.

The cycle of quality improvement can focus on one issue after another as quality problems are tackled and others emerge. A switch in focus may occur at any point – perhaps most likely after the change has been found to have positive effects and other quality issues demand attention. The focus of the clinical audit cycle can, though, stay the same, as would be the case when core standards are continually monitored. Thus the effects of change are monitored, standards are reset at a higher level and the cycle continues. In this case, spiral is a more appropriate metaphor than cycle given the implication of never-ending quality improvement focused upon fixed key aspects of care.

The literature, and also our clinical experience, suggests that implementing change (Stage 5 in Figure 3.1) is the stage of the clinical audit cycle least likely to be carried out. Crombie and Davies (1993) point out that simply recognizing a deficit does not necessarily identify what has to be changed and 'identification of underlying reasons for failure to meet standards' is a missing component of the audit cycle. Their work concerns medical audit but their point is equally relevant to other forms of clinical audit.

The patient care cycle

As with clinical audit, care of individual patients (or other primary care 'units', such as families and patient groups) is often presented as a problem-solving cycle with four key steps:

- assessment
- planning
- implementation
- evaluation.

These steps provide a structure for care delivery and are sometimes used as the basis for other activities, such as documenting care and treatment.

Assessment is likely to involve coming to a diagnosis and might include 'subjective' and 'objective' elements, i.e. the problems or needs of the client as perceived by both the client and the therapist as well as the areas of agreement/disagreement between them. Planning involves goal setting (short- and long-term) and generating treatment plans; evaluation may incorporate specific goal-centred evaluation and more general client review. The patient care cycle is shown in Figure 3.2.

The standards setting cycle

Standards setting may form a semi-independent cycle connected to the clinical audit cycle whether or not health professionals are the main participants in the clinical audit cycle. They may not be closely involved when standards are determined by purchasers (health authorities or GP fundholders), professional organizations or the government acting under initiatives such as the Patient's Charter requirements (Department of Health 1991a) or Health of the Nation targets (Department of Health 1992).

A standards setting cycle is presented in Figure 3.3. In this example, discussion between team members (uni- or multi-professional) in Stage 1 results in the production of draft standards (Stage 2) which are tested for relevance, attainability, clarity and desirability through further discussion in Stage 3; and a final set of standards emerges in Stage 4.

The change cycle

Change might best be represented as a separate cycle outside the clinical audit cycle in circumstances when managers have little involvement in the clinical audit cycle and when quality improvement requires changes that go beyond professional practice to include organizational change.

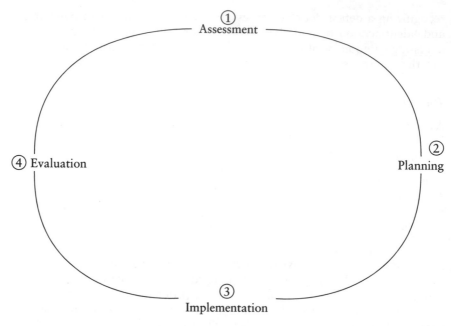

Figure 3.2   The patient care cycle (PCC)

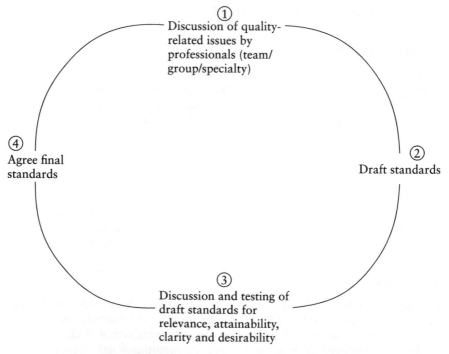

Figure 3.3   The standards setting cycle (SSC)

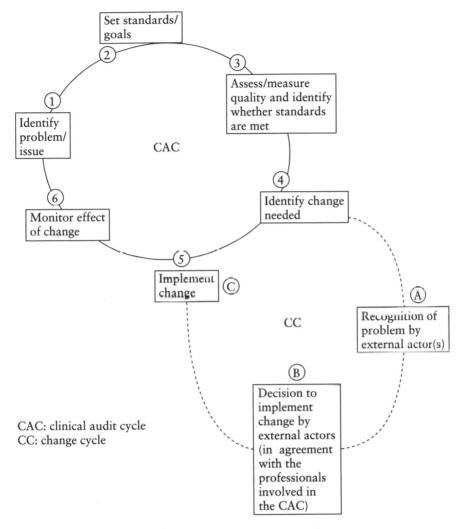

Figure 3.4 The change cycle

Figure 3.4 represents possible stages in a change cycle and its connections with the clinical audit cycle. One example might be that participants
in a clinical audit cycle have found that care falls short of set standards
(Stage 2) and have identified the underlying reason for failure to meet
standards (Stage 3). They discuss this information with managers (or perhaps other professionals) to arouse their concern and alert them to the
need for change. Once a key figure in a senior position recognizes the
problem (Stage A of the change cycle), accepts the proposed diagnosis and
decides to take action (Stage B), planning begins. Planning is likely to

include people who will be involved at the implementation stage (C) and aims to achieve the change in a way that ensures that undesirable impacts on managers and staff are minimized, thus counteracting any effective resistance developing to the proposed change.

The interrogation

We move now to interrogate the cycles; that is to say, are the cycles as we have presented them the best metaphor for describing and understanding clinical audit? The following questions are important:

- are the components of the cycles relevant and complete and the sequences feasible?
- how might the cycles be analysed?
- what links might exist between the clinical audit cycle and the patient care cycle?
- who controls the cycles?
- is the cycle an appropriate metaphor for clinical audit and patient care?

Are the components of the cycles relevant and complete and the sequences feasible?

The clinical audit cycle (Figure 3.1) may be set in motion by one of a number of quality-related initiatives or events, for example, identification of a systems failure (Stage 1), a standards setting initiative (Stage 2), or a quality assessment exercise possibly with standardized tools or measures (Stage 3). Thereafter, different sequences of the cycle seem plausible. A standards setting initiative (Stage 2) may be followed by a quality assessment exercise to identify service deficits (Stage 3). Or Stage 2 may be followed by problem areas being agreed through discussion (Stage 1) rather than by formal assessment and then by changes required being identified (Stage 4). This last example shows that some stages of the cycle may be omitted altogether.

The time available and the effects of different health care services are other variables that will influence the progression and sequence of the clinical audit cycle. For example, surgery has a clear starting point and its effects may be evident within a short time. By contrast mental health interventions often have an uncertain starting point and may show very small effects that are difficult to detect and require a long time-scale for evaluation. These possibilities suggest that the cycle does not always stand up to testing as a chronological or sequential representation of clinical audit, even though it is valuable as a logical representation.

The patient care cycle also comprises a series of components or steps, although in practice the therapist will not always proceed stepwise but will move back and forth around the cycle in response to need. For example, in the case of a mentally disturbed client when cues signifying immediate danger to self or others are observed, a therapist may intervene. In this case intervention has immediately followed assessment of one sign and has by-passed full assessment and diagnosis. In another example, a therapist counselling a patient will continually evaluate the effect of this intervention on the patient and, consequently, may change his or her plans. Although the therapist may omit some stages of the patient care cycle, all stages are likely to be touched upon at least once in the course of any single clinical interaction between therapist and patient.

In this example the patient care cycle is presented as a mental construct with which the therapist monitors his or her performance in the clinical encounter. More often, though, the patient care cycle is used over a longer period and may take many clinical encounters to be completed. For example, a clinical psychologist might assess an elderly person for possible dementia over two clinical sessions and report to a multi-professional team meeting at which a plan of care and treatment is devised in consultation with other health care professionals and the client's relatives. Then the plan might be implemented and progress evaluated in say four weeks time. If this leads to further treatment the cycle starts again and is perhaps best conceived as a spiral around which the patient travels; whether the direction is up or down will depend upon whether the objectives set are met or not.

Components of the patient care cycle do not represent people who have been assessed and are on waiting lists for treatment. Patients may be assessed by one health care professional (e.g. GP) and referred to another (e.g. physiotherapist) for treatment, who may also assess the patient. Alternatively the waiting list could be the topic of the clinical audit cycle. A large pool of potential patients will never access the patient care cycle at all, let alone influence or be influenced by the clinical audit cycle.

The cycle in Figure 3.3 suggests that standards setting is a bottom-up activity in which standards are generated through discussion by a uni- or multi-professional group who may or may not be involved in the associated clinical audit cycle. The standards setting cycle is, though, also influenced by external factors such as the views of patients or of outside bodies. For example, therapists may work from standards produced by professional bodies and adapt these for their local circumstances. In other cases standards setting groups include patients.

Implementing planned change (Stage C in Figure 3.4) should ideally follow the agreed strategic plan and may involve a number of different approaches; for example, further training for people at some levels, building more effective work groups, restructuring the work system and so on. Modifications to the organization may also be agreed including changes to structures and methods and reallocation of resources and responsibilities. Also implemented will be strategies which lead staff to adopt the change; this is generally thought to be best achieved if staff perceive the change as relevant and credible and consistent with their values. In Figure 3.4 movement from the change cycle back into the clinical audit cycle ensures that the change is evaluated.

Stage 2: set standards

Inputs	Process	Outcome
• 10 hours working time	• small group-	• 10 standards statements
• 6 qualified staff = 60 hours	work on values	• therapists reported
• 1 day standards setting	clarification and	improved morale
workshop led by expert	writing standards	
• £100 for computer software	statements	

Figure 3.5 Analysis of Stage 2 of the clinical audit cycle illustrating inputs, process, outcome framework

How might the cycles be analysed?

Understanding clinical audit requires an examination of its different components. One approach to this is to consider inputs, process and outcomes not simply as steps in a chain but as points at each stage of the clinical audit cycle. Analysis of stages of the clinical audit cycle in this way would give us information about the technical aspects of audit (for example, the instruments or methods used to measure quality and the means by which progress towards meeting standards or achieving goals is assessed). It would also give the focus of the audit cycle (on core clinical activities or on activities at different degrees of relatedness to direct patient care).

The input-process-outcome framework might also be applied to stages of the other cycles. Another use of this kind of analysis is represented in Figure 3.5, which illustrates:

• inputs of standards setting (e.g. time, funds and education required)
• the process of standards setting (the procedure involved)
• the outcomes (e.g. ten standards statements were written and the morale of remaining staff was raised).

What links might exist between the clinical audit cycle and the other cycles?

We have applied the metaphor of the cycle to the care of patients and to clinical audit. An important question is to ask how the clinical audit cycle and the patient care cycle might be linked. That is to say, how data from the patient care cycle are picked up in clinical audit and how the results of audit are fed back into the patient care cycle to improve the care that patients receive.

There need not be any direct connection between the patient care cycle and the clinical audit cycle except that any successful clinical audit system will increase the efficiency or effectiveness of the service. For example, an audit of staff training programmes might include staff views and experience but need not consider the care of patients. In other cases information from the care of individual patients will be required in order to assess the quality of aspects of the service as a whole. To take a simple example, a therapist might record in the case notes the time between referral and seeing the patient for the purpose of assessment. If these data are to contribute to clinical audit something must be done with them. They must be collated in some way and be compared against a standard for referral times. In turn, changes in clerical procedures may improve the efficiency of the referral procedure with benefits for the care of patients.

It may be that links between the patient care cycle and the clinical audit cycle become increasingly clear and important as audits focus progressively on core clinical activities. For example, an audit seeking to establish the value of psychotherapy by clinical psychologists, or an occupational therapy programme to increase the independence of institutionalized psychiatric patients, would consider the effects of these core activities on individuals.

If links do exist at which point might the cycles intersect? There are many possible configurations. One example we came across is a mature audit activity, known as the 'individual care programme' and developed by Perkins *et al.* (1992), which had completed one audit cycle and embarked on another. It also had successfully linked the patient care cycle to the clinical audit cycle.

This multi-professional mental health unit had developed a system to measure long-term clients' individual outcomes in terms of functioning, quality of care and quality of life. Each client had an individual care programme which was reviewed twice yearly. New standards were set for the following six months. The client was involved in the setting and review of goals.

Standardized instruments were used to evaluate the quality of care. On the basis of scores achieved, discussions focused on how best to improve the quality of care that was wanting. Then each team set itself specific targets for change over a defined period (six months) and these targets were audited using a goal-attainment scale. Measurements were repeated using the same instruments. The results were discussed when targets were reviewed and new targets were set.

Data to assess the target outcomes were collected on a continuous basis by the rehabilitation teams. Recording methods relating to each target were in place. For example, quantitative data would be collected to meet a patient's target to decrease her incontinence. The normal recording practice of the rehabilitation teams was to record patients' behaviour with reference to their individual care plans. Data were collected manually, often by nursing staff at shift handovers, and were then computerized.

The teams were also trying to work out how best to involve users more in the audit process. Clients had participated in setting targets during discussions held separately from those with the staff so that there was no possibility of influence or intimidation. Some targets would be set by staff and others by users. Clients were also involved in auditing whether the targets had been achieved.

The professionals felt that this audit system improved care and brought about noticeable change. They identified two points as important in achieving change: involve all relevant staff and users in the change; and make sure that everyone knows and understands exactly what the aims are – that is to say, the goals must be precise and achievable.

Change was measured quantitatively (on entry to the scheme and at six-monthly intervals) through:

- individually programmed treatment and care outcomes
- ward management practices
- contact with the community
- the physical environment.

Of the eleven team targets specified, improvement on nine of them was noted after six months.

Figure 3.6 shows the audit process followed in this example as two interconnected audit spirals: the providers' spiral and the users' spiral. The two spirals are independent yet closely connected and make contact at certain points. For example, users met as a group and discussed the quality of the service without input from staff (Point 3) so avoiding contamination of views, but there were times when staff and users got together to set targets for change (Point 4). Targets set by users and targets set by staff were evaluated independently by users as well as by staff (Point 6).

Links between the clinical audit cycle and factors both within and outside the provider unit are discussed in Chapter 6. We have shown some links between individual patient outcomes and audit outcomes in Chapter 4.

Who controls the cycles?

The question of control is likely to influence the shape and scope of audit and the potential of the clinical audit cycle to effect changes in practice which will have benefits for patient care. An important question is whether clinical audit is under the control of health care professionals or of management. The contribution by managers ranges from minimal intervention to explicit control, in which the professional is required to adopt a designated approach. At this end of the scale clinical audit is driven by management in such a way that results would directly affect rewards for the professionals involved.

The power of clinical audit to make quality improvements is likely to be constrained by the membership of the clinical audit group because they will, naturally enough, want to discuss areas over which they have control. It seems probable therefore, that clinical audit cycles in which managers are either excluded or only have limited influence will be confined to implementing changes only in relation to professional practice. On the other hand, clinical audit cycles in which managers are more influential may also seek organizational change. If managers are not involved in the clinical audit cycle but organizational change is needed, then this change

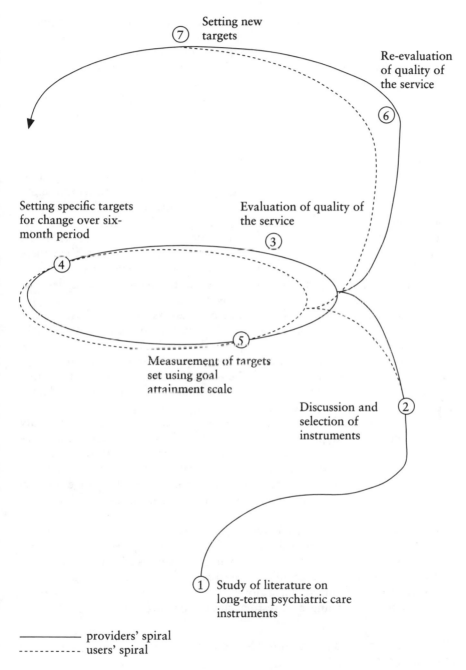

Figure 3.6 The individual care programme: providers' and users' spirals

will have to be achieved outside the clinical audit cycle. So, for example, it may require members of the clinical audit group selling the need for change to managers and thereby kick-starting a change cycle.

The discussion so far has identified professionals or managers as key players in the clinical audit cycle. But there are other important stakeholders who may be directly involved and be more or less influential. In particular, purchasers are increasingly taking responsibility for funding clinical audit. Another question is the effect on clinical audit of being controlled by professional heads who are also service managers.

The patient care cycle might be owned by the professional or shared with the patient depending upon the degree of collaboration between the professional and the patient in planning and delivering care and treatment. It might also be uni- or multi-professional, according to involvement by more than one discipline in the treatment programme, and it might involve inter-agency collaboration. If more than one professional group is involved and each monitors the effects of their contribution on the patient, then there would be several patient care cycles for each patient, some uni- and others multi-professional. Whether this is reflected in the patient's notes depends on whether the professions keep their own record or contribute to a single multi-professional record of the patient's progress. Current emphasis on systems of case management and key working within community health care settings and the rise of consumerism raises the possibility of increasing numbers of patient care cycles which are the product of inter-professional and inter-agency collaboration to which the patient makes a major contribution.

A question relevant to ownership of the change cycle is whether change induced by management is compatible with the philosophy of clinical audit. An example might be an executive decision made to impose a new duty rota system to ensure patients 24-hour-a-day access to services. Customary approaches to effecting change include re-educating staff to overcome resistance based on poor information, facilitating staff to overcome their resistance by reducing the natural anxiety associated with change, or persuading them to accept the change by instilling enthusiasm for what could be achieved.

Crombie and Davies (1993) see approaches to change such as feeding back information on current practice and issuing general management guidelines to all staff as limited in their effectiveness. They advocate detailed guidance on specific topics to staff who need it most based upon an analysis of why standards have not been achieved. This guidance may be the basis for developing and testing clinical or care protocols.

How far is the cycle an appropriate metaphor for clinical audit and patient care?

As a logical representation of clinical audit, the cycle seems to be of value; although probably the spiral metaphor is more appropriate, particularly when continuous quality improvement is emphasized.

As we have noted, the clinical audit cycle might be disrupted at the point of carrying out change to improve practice although there could be second-order effects which are unplanned and unanticipated (e.g. improved staff morale, improved communications, raised awareness of the need for audit). Clinical audit can also be applied to a single activity like setting standards. These patterns of clinical audit raise questions about the value of the cycle as a realistic representation of audit practice; in some cases clinical audit might be better represented as several stages on a straight line rather than as a cycle.

We cannot be sure that the patient care cycle is a realistic representation of patient care and treatment. The cycle might be used as a framework for analysing practitioner–patient interaction but it is far from certain that the practitioner consciously follows anything approximating a cycle during the process of interaction with patients. Indeed, there is some evidence that expert practitioners are guided by intuition and experience in their inter-action with patients and find it more difficult than novices to articulate the reasons behind their actions (Benner 1984).

Similarly it is uncertain how far the components of the patient care cycle reflect the experience of most patients. Take, for example, a patient who is referred to the physiotherapist for treatment of back pain, is prescribed a course of six sessions, attends two treatments, cancels his next appoint-ment and does not attend again. Here assessment is followed by planning and the start of implementation. There is no evaluation and the patient is discharged. In this example the course of care and treatment is episodic rather than continuous and might be better represented as linear rather than cyclical.

It is likely to be the case that some patients receive individually planned treatment whereas others, in certain diagnostic categories, receive a treat-ment package influenced by a clinical protocol. For patients who receive standard packages the patient care cycle might not be relevant. Thus questions are raised about the cycle as an appropriate metaphor for under-standing the care of all patients.

With respect to standards setting it might be that standards are simply passed on to health care professionals by managers. If this is the case, using a cycle to represent the sequence of standards setting is inappropri-ate. Even when groups of professionals develop standards in consultation with users, different sequences of the stages are possible. So we can see that, as with the clinical audit cycle and the patient care cycle, the stand-ards setting cycle does not stand up to scrutiny as a chronological sequence in every case.

Turning finally to the change cycle, some authorities note the limitations of the cyclical model as an adequate representation of the change process. Studies of organizational change show that it is not always planned – in the sense of specifying objectives and methods and progressing along an agreed route – nor does it follow a logical sequence (e.g. McLean *et al.* 1982; Lovelady 1983). Rather, change processes vary and are contingent on organizational needs and circumstances. Change agents might be better described as creating change through innovative intervention activities carried out on an *ad hoc* basis in the light of reappraisals throughout the change process.

The process of analysis we developed from this framework of cycles (patient care, standards setting, clinical audit and change) is explained with worked examples in the annex to Chapter 5.

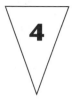

4 / The nature of clinical audit and progress made

Anémone Kober

This chapter provides a flavour of the audit culture and stock of audit activities as they have been and are now taking place. As we shall see, they vary considerably because 'the professions included have very different histories, have different balances between different client groups, and operate with different timescales' (Normand *et al.* 1991b).

We show the merits of multi-professional compared to uni-professional clinical audit and progress made on outcome measurement and elements of structure. In conclusion, we identify some implications for the development of clinical audit for the four professions. Audit developments in clinical psychology, occupational therapy, physiotherapy and speech and language therapy are described in Appendices 3 and 4.

Intra- and inter-professional audit activity

What kind of audit activities are now taking place? From a search of correspondence from the then active National Nursing and Therapy Audit Network, its first six newsletters (1992–3) and the Clearing House database (January 1994), a crude count of audit activities within the four professions is given in Table 4.1.

This gives only a rough idea of reported audit activity; many more projects will not have reached the sources searched. However, of the 61 uni-professional audit projects reported in the two-year period, most were initiated by physiotherapists or speech and language therapists and fewest by clinical psychologists. Bearing in mind the number of therapists employed in each profession – speech and language therapy is a third the size of occupational therapy and a quarter the size of physiotherapy, and clinical psychology is much the smallest of the four (Devore Associates 1993)

Table 4.1   Audit activities within the four professions

Uni-professional audit activities	
clinical psychology	9
occupational therapy	13
physiotherapy	18
speech and language therapy	21
Total	61
Multi-professional audit activities	38

– speech and language therapists seem, from this information, to be particularly active in audit.

Most of the projects are classified as outcome studies that usually involved evaluation of the effects on clients of therapeutic intervention or of the service more generally. The multi-professional audit projects were carried out by different combinations of the four professions, with or without other professions; of the four professions it was occupational therapists and physiotherapists who most often worked together.

It may be that clinical psychologists use research journals more frequently than the other professions to publish their work and so choose not to use the sources searched here. A data source of audit activities in clinical psychology in England and Wales is the British Psychological Society's Standing Advisory Committee's Stocktake of Audit Projects (Berger 1994, personal communication). This database is still in preparation and, when we consulted it, its last entry was dated March 1994. It contains 97 entries of which some two-thirds appear to involve clinical psychologists only and one-third could be described as multi-professional. A crude count revealed 17 audit activities that might be classified as structure-based, 24 process, 37 outcome, 14 process-outcome and 5 activities that cover all three of Donabedian's categories.

Another database of audit activities within the therapy professions has recently been published (Department of Health 1994c). This is the report of the three-year programme of audit in nursing and therapy professions supported by the Department of Health. The database reveals that 456 nursing and therapy audit activities were funded by the 14 regions in England in 1992–3. As a conservative estimate, 81 (18 per cent) of these activities involved one or more of the therapy professions. Only those activities that specified at least one of the four professions (i.e. clinical psychology, occupational therapy, physiotherapy, speech and language therapy) were counted; we could not be certain that activities specifying 'the therapy professions' or 'professions allied to medicine' included one of these four.

Of the 81 audit activities, 21 (26 per cent) were uni-professional and 60 (74 per cent) multi-professional. Clinical psychologists were involved in 15 of these, occupational therapists in 33, physiotherapists in 43 and speech and language therapists in 24. Bearing in mind the size of the professions, it seems that speech and language therapists and clinical psychologists are particularly active in audit proportionate to their numbers.

The nursing and therapy database shows clearly that the proportion of uni- to multi-professional audit activities has reversed with three-quarters now multi-professional, thus reflecting the centrally initiated drive to promote multi-professional clinical audit. There has also been a shift in the focus of audit; we estimate that 19 of the 81 activities are structure-based, 18 are process, 16 outcome, 6 process-outcome and 16 include structure, process and outcome elements (the few remaining we could not classify). It does seem that the move towards multi-professional audit, actively promoted by the NHS Executive, has encouraged more structure and process audit activity than before.

The audit funding initiative by the Department of Health since 1991 has unleashed considerable talent amongst the therapy professions in introducing clinical audit activities and submitting bids for funding. The requirement from the start seems to have been for multi-professional audit, unlike the much greater separate funding earmarked exclusively for medical audit. From 1994 the funds available have been combined into one allocation with no distinction between medical audit and the rest, with interesting effects on how the cake is divided locally. The recommendation by the Department of Health that funds are used to advance multi-professional clinical audit might encourage the medical profession to take the lead, either by facilitating and collaborating in clinical audit in a collegial teamworking approach, or by taking control and colonizing clinical audit activities across the therapy and nursing professions as well as its own. However, the Department of Health makes clear that: 'no specific professional group should be seen as the natural leader of clinical audit and all health professionals should have the opportunity to obtain relevant skills in auditing. Training resources should be equally accessible to all' (Department of Health 1994a). This robust statement offers a mandate to the health professions in their pursuit of useful clinical audit.

Classification of audit in the four health professions

Here we describe the categories of audit activities, methods, data used and outcome measurement we have seen. We look at the nature of audit (uni- or multi-professional or both) and present views on outcome measures, and on the feasibility and desirability of a common framework for clinical audit.

Modes of classification

We have classified the audit activities according to Donabedian's structure, process and outcome framework and our own definitions of clinical audit.

As we have described in Chapter 1, Donabedian's categories answer the following questions:

- what facilities are available? (structure)
- what treatment/care is given? (process)
- what is the result for the patient? (outcome).

Our own categories of clinical audit are core clinical activity, closely associated activity and less closely associated activity. To reiterate, core clinical activities are identified as a process concerned with the assessment of clinical activities directly related to patients with a view to making a judgement on the quality of *care* delivered. Closely associated and less closely associated clinical audit activities are concerned with the assessment of activities associated with the treatment of patients, with a view to making judgements on the quality of the *services* delivered.

Table 4.2 presents the range of audit activities we have seen. Audit activities can belong to more than one category (core clinical, closely associated or less closely associated) and can focus on one or more of the structure, process and outcome categories.

The number of audit activities within each category was roughly equal: core clinical (51), closely associated (58) and less closely associated (54). More activities focused on the process of care (106) than on outcome and/or structure (57 each). Thus, more than two-thirds of the audit activities were linked to process. Some therapists saw a natural history, or chronology, of audit in these professions in which process is tackled before outcome.

The four professions led a similar number of audit activities: 34 were led by physiotherapists, 33 by clinical psychologists, 31 by occupational therapists and 27 by speech and language therapists.

Occupational therapists were involved in somewhat more activities than the other three professions (55 compared to 33 for clinical psychologists, 41 for physiotherapists and 38 for speech and language therapists). As for professions other than our four, nurses were involved in 33 of the activities, doctors in 28, dieticians in 3 and other professionals in 9. Nursing and medicine were the professions most likely to be involved in multi-professional audit with the four professions.

Twice as many of the audit activities were uni-professional (89) rather than multi-professional (46).

The structure, process or outcome focus of uni- and multi-professional audit activities are presented in Table 4.3. A slightly greater proportion of uni- (49 per cent) than multi-professional activities (46 per cent) were related to process. And a slightly greater proportion of multi-professional (29 per cent) than uni-professional activities (24 per cent) relate to structure. Overall, however, these differences are negligible.

Table 4.4 shows that only 28 per cent of the uni-professional audit activities were related to core clinical issues compared to 36 per cent of the multi-professional activities. By contrast, a greater percentage of uni-

Table 4.2 Range of audit activities investigated in the six main sites

Site	Nature			Category*				Focus*			Profession(s) leading*					Professions involved*							
	Uni	Multi	Total	Clinical audit 1	Clinical audit 2	Clinical audit 3	Other	Struc-ture	Pro-cess	Out-come	CP	OT	PT	SLT	Other	CP	OT	PT	SLT	Diet-etics	Nurs-ing	Medi-cine	Other
Site 1	10	4	14	7	7	4	–	5	10	7	–	4	6	3	1	–	7	9	5	1	3	3	1
Site 2	41	18	59	21	19	25	3	28	44	35	12	16	19	11	1	16	24	17	15	2	12	9	6
Site 3	14	1	15	8	10	3	–	2	13	6	3	3	4	4	1	2	2	3	3	–	1	–	1
Site 4	3	3	6	1	5	3	–	3	5	1	–	2	5	–	1	–	5	6	–	–	1	–	–
Site 5	10	6	16	4	11	7	–	7	12	2	–	–	–	9	5	–	6	6	15	–	6	6	1
Site 6	11	14	25	10	6	12	–	12	22	5	13	6	–	–	8	15	11	–	–	–	10	10	–
Total	89	46	135	51	58	54	3	57	106	57	33	31	34	27	17	33	55	41	38	3	33	28	9

* Audit activities in these sections can belong to more than one category

Clinical audit 1: audit of core clinical activities
Clinical audit 2: audit of closely associated activities
Clinical audit 3: audit of less closely associated activities

CP: clinical psychology
OT: occupational therapy
PT: physiotherapy
SLT: speech and language therapy

Table 4.3 Uni- and multi-professional audit activities by focus (structure, process or outcome) (percentages in parentheses)

	Structure*	Process*	Outcome*	Total
Uni-professional	35 (24)	71 (49)	38 (26)	144 (100)
Multi-professional	22 (29)	35 (46)	19 (25)	76 (100)
Total	57 (26)	106 (48)	57 (26)	220 (100)

* Audit activities in these sections can belong to more than one category

Table 4.4 Uni- and multi-professional audit activities by category (core, closely associated or less closely associated) (percentages in parentheses)

	Clinical audit (core)*	Clinical audit (closely associated)*	Clinical audit closely associated)*	Other	Total
Uni-professional	32 (28)	43 (38)	36 (31)	3 (3)	114 (100)
Multi-professional	19 (36)	15 (29)	18 (35)		52 (100)
Total	51 (31)	58 (35)	54 (32)	3 (2)	166 (100)

* Audit activities in these sections can belong to more than one category

professional activities concerned closely associated activities (38 per cent) than was the case with multi-professional audit (29 per cent). And roughly similar percentages of uni- and multi-professional activities (31 and 35 per cent respectively) were concerned with less closely associated activities.

These findings indicate that, contrary to a commonly held view, multi-professional audit was at least as likely as uni-professional audit to tackle core clinical issues. Moreover the audit activities investigated related largely to the process of care, whether they were uni- or multi-professional.

The audit topics

Figures 4.1 and 4.2 summarize the nature of the audit topics we have seen according to structure, process and outcome and our three categories of clinical audit.

Methods used for audit

Methods of audit described in the literature and used in the activities were:

• case presentation
• peer review

Structure
- environmental and equipment audit
- standards setting
- caseload analysis and monitoring
- client prioritization
- individual care programme
- computerization of individual patient plans and care outcomes
- role overlap between professions and generic working

Process
- service agreements with purchasers
- standards setting
- access to services
- audit of referral procedures
- improper referrals and 'did not attend' audit
- case note audit
- multidisciplinary case review
- client prioritization
- needs assessment of patients/clients
- individual care programme and case management (peer review)
- shared action planning
- special interest group audits (e.g. chest problems, osteoarthritis of knee, spina bifida)
- intervention programmes
- discharge procedures
- achievement of standards/goals
- identification of unmet clinical service demands
- external audit of all services against process and organizational standards
- individual performance review
- clinical supervision

Outcome
- standards setting
- outcome measures and outcomes of care (e.g. spina bifida, osteoarthritis of knee, out-patients, young physically disabled, learning disabilities, stroke unit)
- clinical baseline for conversational skills
- patient/client and referrer satisfaction

Figure 4.1 Audit topics classified according to structure, process and outcome

- adverse events and sentinel events
- criteria-based audit
- surveys of patients, referrers and/or clients.

We found criteria-based audits to be by far the most common, followed by surveys, case presentations and peer review, and least common were adverse and/or sentinel events. The material that follows contains information about each of these audit methods and illustrative examples drawn from what we have seen in the health professions.

Core clinical activities
- standards setting
- special interest group audit (e.g. chest problems, osteoarthritis of knee, footwear, cognitive therapy)
- outcome measures and outcomes of care (e.g. physical rehabilitation, stroke patients with dysphasia, young physically disabled, spina bifida, memory clinic, incidents of self-harm, hand therapy)
- client and referrer satisfaction
- information for stroke patients and their carers
- peer review of client programmes
- multidisciplinary case review and case management (peer review)
- case note audit
- computerization of individual patient plans and care outcomes

Closely associated activities
- standards setting
- needs assessment of a mental health rehabilitation service
- case records audit (peer review)
- case management audit (peer review)
- audit of referring agents
- individual performance review
- equality of access to services
- identification of unmet clinical service demands
- role overlap and generic working

Less closely associated activities
- standards setting
- service agreements with purchasers
- patient prioritization
- individual care programme
- caseload analysis
- discharge monitoring
- environmental and equipment audit
- review of out-patients' waiting lists
- individual performance review
- training needs of staff

Figure 4.2 Audit topics classified into core, closely associated and less closely associated categories

Case presentation
This involves the review of individual cases. Review of randomly selected cases can be repetitive and time consuming and so presentations focusing on particular topics are more popular and educational (Crombie *et al.* 1993). An advantage of this method is its simplicity. A disadvantage is that usually only a small number of cases can be assessed and the process is subjective.

We found case presentation to be fairly common, either as part of an individual supervision session or as a method of peer review with a larger group. A feature of this method is that it enables health professionals to communicate effectively with each other and share ideas and practices. However, if the team atmosphere is tense, case presentations can increase the stress of staff in team meetings. Also, as a community psychiatric nurse told us, 'there is a tendency to personalize issues and achievements do not always last'. On the other hand, case presentations to a group of peers can encourage therapists to keep their standards high. Case presentation is a means of addressing complex moral issues that can get overlooked with quantitative audit methods.

Example

Topic:	Case presentation in clinical psychology, which included all specialities in a health authority.
Category and focus:	Core clinical activity linked to the process of care.
Aim:	Developmental and educational.
Method:	Weekly or fortnightly meetings of specialty groups. Each clinical psychologist would present approximately two cases per year selected at random. A protocol for these case presentations had been set. There was a list of points and questions in key areas to address during each presentation. The method could also be described as a structured peer review.
Outcome:	Goals and action points were identified and there was a follow-up to check that action points were put into practice.

Peer review

Peer review describes audits in which one group of professionals visits a similar group in a different district, hospital or region (Firth-Cozens 1993). It qualifies as audit if definite standards are set and procedures are systematic.

We found that a clear distinction was not always made between peer review and case presentation. Both were used to describe presentation of a case. The two examples below were described to us as peer review.

Example 1

Topic:	Structured peer review in clinical psychology (learning disabilities).
Category and focus:	Core clinical and closely associated activity related to process and outcome.
Aims:	Review specific cases, improve care, develop and educate staff.
Method:	The psychologist checked that various steps of the process of care had been accomplished. A checklist

	with a series of questions had been devised and was answered for each case (e.g. was enough time spent on the case? How was the care recorded in the notes? Was any important aspect of care omitted?).
Outcome:	A negative outcome was the length of time required to fill in the checklists and prepare the case. This meant that few cases per clinical psychologist were presented.

Example 2

Topic:	Peer review in speech and language therapy. The definition of peer review used by this service was: 'A frank discussion between two or more colleagues of the same grade, without fear of criticism, regarding the quality of care provided against agreed standards, in a context which allows for evolutionary change in standards. It should lead to "action" where practice has not matched agreed standards, so the quality of care is improved' (Enderby *et al.* 1992).
Category and focus:	Core clinical and closely associated activity related to process and outcome.
Aim:	Improve case notes and case management.
Method:	Therapists met once a year to present two self-selected cases each. They also took five case notes at random from each other's files and checked the contents against a predetermined checklist. The checklists were sent to the audit coordinator for collation and a brief report was given to the professional service manager.

Outcomes and changes required:

- The audit of case notes was time consuming and did not require clinical skills. It was planned to delegate this part of the peer review to clerical staff
- a protocol was being drawn up specifying items that should be covered during the case management peer review
- it was decided that in future peer review would take place among peers of the same specialty in existing support groups, even if therapists were not of the same grade
- it is important to define action following peer review clearly so that therapists see there is a point to such activity

- colleagues who share knowledge in the same specialty should be involved (statement of intent to move into multi-professional audit)
- it is essential to trust each other and respect confidentiality during the peer review process
- 'multiple reviewers' should be involved in the peer review process rather than just one other peer.

In this example, peer review was moving from closely associated clinical activities to core clinical activities. The activities that involved monitoring the process of care (e.g. extracting information from notes) were being delegated to clerical staff. The educational, formative element of peer review had not so far been prominent but it was planned to give this more emphasis.

Adverse and sentinel events

Adverse event review examines examples of poor care and outcome; sentinel or critical events are examples of serious adverse events. We have seen few audits using this method although one example is described.

Example

Topic:	Incidents of self-harm in a mental health community unit.
Category and focus:	Core clinical audit related to process and outcome.
Aim:	To identify what could have helped to prevent or anticipate the incident.
Methods:	Two multidisciplinary mental health teams worked together reviewing the case notes of patients who had harmed themselves; random case reviews and checks of case notes took place to see whether care plans had been completed and if minimal requirements had been fulfilled (named day worker, clear care plan, medication recorded).
Outcome:	Problems in relation to cases were identified but it is unclear whether this brought about any real change.

Criteria-based audit

Criteria-based audits define specific criteria that can be compared to actual practice either prospectively or retrospectively. The criteria specifying good care are usually developed during discussions among clinicians (Crombie *et al.* 1993). It is common to define the optimum level of quality of care or the best possible outcome.

Most of the audits we have seen are criteria-based in one form or another. Criteria were set either before the audit or as part of it. In many cases, the audits were still at the stage of setting standards against which outcomes of care are audited.

Example 1

Topic:	Audit of the quality of reports in speech and language therapy.
Category and focus:	Closely associated audit activity related to process.
Aim:	Standardize and improve the content of reports.
Methods:	• The current state of the reports was examined by a principal therapist (e.g. the way the reports were written, what items were included, format) • an open forum including all the therapists involved led to the identification of guidelines about how to write reports • every three months or so the principal audited all the reports in her section against these guidelines.
Outcome:	Some improvement identified but not measured.

Example 2

Topic:	Audit of patients' records in occupational therapy and physiotherapy.
Category and focus:	Closely associated audit activity related to process.
Aim:	Improve the quality of records. The standards of patients' records had been identified as low during an external service review carried out by the district health authority's quality office.
Methods:	• A questionnaire survey of occupational therapists and physiotherapists was carried out to identify existing practice • discussions followed analysis of the data and problem areas were identified • a new record form was devised • new standards for record keeping and referrals were set up • random audit of patients' records using the new form was carried out.
Outcome:	The audit showed an improvement in the quality of patients' records.

Example 3

Topic:	Computerized caseload analysis.
Category and focus:	Closely associated audit activity related to structure and outcome.
Aim:	Monitor specific client groups and the number of clients seen by therapists.

Method: Number and type of clients seen by each therapist
                     was monitored regularly. Information was made
                     available to each therapist in the form of monthly
                     computer print-outs, pie charts and diagrams.

Outcome: It was felt that presenting this type of information
                     to each therapist on a regular basis was sufficient
                     to bring about improvements.

Example 4

Topic: Outcomes of care in a rehabilitation hospital ward
                     (head injury).

Category and focus: Core clinical audit activity related to outcome.

Aim: Measure the outcome for each patient in the ward
                     fortnightly and at discharge.

Methods: • Meetings were led by the consultant and cases
                       were presented by senior registrars, but all
                       professions involved with the care were included
                       (speech and language therapy, occupational
                       therapy, physiotherapy, nursing). This was an
                       example of medical audit moving into multi-
                       professional clinical audit
                     • short-term and long-term goals were set on
                       admission for each patient
                     • at discharge, outcomes were plotted for each
                       patient using a scale measuring levels of
                       independence, and entry scores were compared
                       to exit scores
                     • goals set on admission were checked. A
                       discussion of each case followed
                     • about ten patients were reviewed at each
                       fortnightly meeting.

Outcome: The team planned to devise a new scale that
                     would include other patient outcomes.

Example 5

Topic: Individual care programme for long-term clients in
                     a mental health rehabilitation ward.

Category and focus: All three categories of clinical audit with an
                     emphasis on core clinical audit activities related to
                     outcome, process and structure.

Aim: Measure individual care outcomes.

Methods: • The multidisciplinary team had developed a
                       system to measure individual client outcomes in
                       terms of functioning, quality of care and quality
                       of life

- twice-yearly review of each client's individual care programme
- new standards were set for the next six months. The client was involved in the setting and review of goals.

Outcome: The measurements showed improvements in care and noticeable change.

Surveys

Surveys carried out by questionnaire or interview are often used to measure outcome. They require time, expertise and funds. Postal surveys are liable to low response rates and, as for all questionnaire surveys, bias in the form of the 'halo' effect can occur (Fitzpatrick 1991a, 1991b). We found questionnaire surveys to be a popular means of assessing satisfaction of patients, carers and other customers (e.g. referrers, general practitioners). They were often small scale and are not checked for reliability and validity.

Example

Topic: Audit of referring agents.

Category and focus: Closely associated and less closely associated clinical audit related to structure and process.

Aim: Improve waiting times and communication between speech and language therapists and referrers.

Method: Pilot study involved sending a range of questionnaires to therapists and various referrers to find out who referred to whom; questionnaires were sent to referrers asking about various areas of the speech and language therapy service (e.g. questions on waiting times).

Outcome: The audit had occurred twice. The information from the questionnaire survey was used to audit the standards of the speech and language therapy department (for instance waiting time between referral and first appointment). This audit was led by the professional service manager. Results were reported in writing to the care group manager and chief executive.

Instruments used often included interview and questionnaire schedules with patients, carers or health professionals as ways of obtaining information on existing practices and seeking views on desirable changes. It was not unusual to come across other instruments devised by the therapists or audit coordinators such as:

- goal attainment scales and measurement scales, or adaptation of existing scales

- checklists
- protocols of care/treatment
- assessment forms/discharge forms/various audit forms.

The time and effort spent in devising and applying these instruments can be considerable. There is a real issue as to whether therapists have the time and skills necessary to devise complex scales and questionnaire schedules.

Progress in outcome assessment in the therapy professions

We have seen some coherence of audit development in the sense that there was progress from what was regarded by many therapists as the easier audit activities relating to structure and process towards what was perceived as the more difficult audit of outcome. There was often, too, a progression from standards setting to auditing. There is no doubt that outcome measurement is seen as extremely difficult for professions whose clients have long-term protracted ill-health. Clinical psychologists and occupational therapists made this point particularly strongly.

We have sought out examples that demonstrate whether assessment of outcomes of care, used as part of evaluation of the patient care process, were merged into broader clinical audit outcome measures. What follows is a description of approaches to outcome assessment that we have seen used and examples of activities that managed to link patient care evaluation to a wider clinical audit endeavour.

Standardized scales for individual outcome measurement

Measurement of individual outcomes of care at the patient's discharge from hospital is part of therapists' normal practice. Many extended this to include interim outcome measurement at periods during treatment as well as at discharge.

Standardized scales and measures were used as part of patient assessment and evaluation of care and treatment at the discretion of the therapist. Commonly used scales included activities of daily living scales (e.g. the Barthel Index) health status measures (e.g. the Nottingham Health Profile, the General Health Questionnaire), anxiety and depression scales (e.g. the Hospital and Anxiety Scale, the Beck Depression Inventory) and communication tests (e.g. the Reynard Test).

Occupational therapists, particularly, felt that outcome measurement using standard scales has limitations. They are time consuming to complete and often yield less satisfactory results than more subjective methods, like a discussion with the patient or carers. As one told us, 'OT is about using your relationship with the client and using your personality and it is individualistic ... OTs are specifically looking at quite elusive areas, things like motivation or quality of life of the client.'

A major problem for all the professions is the difficulty of specifying outcomes that result from specific interventions. Also, quantitative measurement of outcome is difficult with some client groups, such as people with learning disabilities.

Goal setting

Goal setting is a common way of measuring individual outcomes of care. This usually involves writing in the patient's notes at the onset of the episode of care what the problems are, what the goals of treatment are, and the date for monitoring whether these goals are achieved. With some client groups and for some professions goal setting is easy. With a stroke patient, for example, a physiotherapy goal might be that the patient will achieve chair-to-bed transfer independently without assistance within two weeks. A measurement scale of, say, one to five might be used by the therapist to rate the level of independence reached by the patient.

Quantitative goal measurement was not always appropriate, however. Some patients' notes contained a description of whether the aims of treatment had been met at the time of discharge from hospital. These qualitative entries were used as outcome assessments.

User involvement

Generally speaking, it is considered useful to include the patient's views in goal setting because it encourages professionals and patients to consider each other's expectations and objectives. Many of the problems of dissatisfaction with treatment and outcome occur because patients and professionals have different expectations of treatment.

In a learning disabilities service, the clinical psychologists were trying to determine the patients' rather than their own goals. Goals were negotiated with the patient, identifying the areas where the clinical psychologists could help and those where they could not. At the end of each session, the therapist assessed whether the aims had been reached. This involved outcome and process measurement; interim outcomes at the end of each session were fed into the final outcome picture. It was the case, though, that the patients were involved only at the goal setting phase.

In a physiotherapy service, the patient's opinion was taken into account in care planning. Two computerized databases coexisted: the subjective database (what the patient said about his condition), and the objective database (the assessment made by the therapist).

Goals of treatment were agreed with the patient and assessed by the therapists. Again, the patient was not directly involved in the assessment and evaluation and this could have serious ethical implications (an unscrupulous therapist could make sure that the outcome was positive, for example).

Multi-professional outcome assessment

In our experience, multi-professional outcome measurement is still at an early stage. There seems to be little compatibility between outcome measures used by different clinicians in the health professions generally. Linking non-medical clinical audit and medical audit is in its infancy. Some therapists maintained that their outcome measures are unlikely to be compatible with those used in medicine because therapists are concerned mainly with the measurement of handicap, and doctors with impairment. There was enthusiasm, however, to find outcome measures that can be used effectively by the different professions so that global patient outcomes can be measured and passed on to purchasers.

Individual patient outcomes can, in the opinion of many therapists, be quite easily measured in a multi-professional way. One way of doing this was explained to us. Each profession sets goals and rates the expected outcome depending on specific criteria relevant to each. The multi-professional team meets and establishes the problems for each patient. Goals are set for each problem. These goals are discussed with the patient and evaluated at the end of treatment. The steps, therefore, are:

- group discussion (including the patient) to identify the patient's problems and needs
- establishing common goals
- measuring goals at completion of treatment.

Each profession first assesses if they have met their individual goals, after which the multi-professional goals are assessed.

In another example, a multi-professional rehabilitation team had done considerable work in setting up a system to measure multi-professional outcomes of care.

Example

Topic:	Multi-professional outcomes of care in a rehabilitation hospital ward (head injury).
Category and focus:	Core clinical audit activity and measurement of outcome.
Aim:	Measure the outcome for each patient in the ward at discharge. Meetings occurred fortnightly. All professions involved with the care were included: speech and language therapists, occupational therapists, physiotherapists, doctors and nurses. This was an example of medical-initiated audit that had moved into multi-professional clinical audit.
Methods:	• Short-term and long-term goals were set on admission for each patient

- at discharge outcomes were plotted for each patient using a scale measuring levels of independence. Entry score was compared to exit score
- goals met were checked against goals set on admission and a discussion of each case followed. Each case was presented by a senior registrar and discussed by the consultant with input from others in the team
- about ten patients were reviewed at each meeting (fortnightly).

Criticism of the system was that the scale was too general to replace the normal assessment and evaluation that each health professional would carry out. For example, only one question in the multi-professional scale was related to communication and so was insufficient to assess the speech and language therapist's input. This problem would be remedied, however, by combining specific, highly specialized uni-professional outcome scales with broader multi-professional scales.

This initiative had moved successfully into multi-professional clinical audit. The project related to all stages of the patient care cycle – assessment, planning, implementation and evaluation. The challenge this team now faced was how to move from individual patient outcome measurement to service outcome measurement required for clinical audit. It is to assessment of the service that we now turn.

Service outcome assessment

We have seen few examples of service outcome measurement. We do not underestimate the difficulties of moving from the measurement of individual outcomes of care to service outcome measurement.

Satisfaction questionnaire surveys of patients, carers or referrers are often the only form of service outcome measure used. Such questionnaires are limited as outcome measures because clients tend to be unduly grateful for the service received and have low expectations of what could be done for them. Referrers may also be reluctant to criticize, particularly if they can relinquish a problem to someone else.

A minority view was that introducing service outcome measures increases professionals' workload. One therapist told us that service outcome measures would be accepted only if they saved time or if they were imposed by managers.

Generally speaking, though, service outcome measures were considered to be a crucial issue but were as yet under-developed because of their complexity. Again, the concept of a natural history of audit is useful. Tackling process issues of audit first was seen as logical, before moving into outcomes: 'nothing has been done on outcomes. We're very interested in it, but very little has been done in the formal sense of audit. We felt it was more important to look at process within the time-scale available (six months)' (senior physiotherapist).

Although little headway had been made in moving from the stage of individual outcome measurement to auditing service outcomes, many therapists saw the potential to making links between the care of individual patients and clinical audit. In the words of a therapist: 'it works two ways, I suppose. In one way you're looking at the effectiveness of treatment for the individual clients building up to a knowledge base of treatment of specific disorders . . . something which is extremely effective with one client might not be with another, which in turn leads to questions about the effectiveness of the whole service.'

In this service, the therapists were involved in case presentations of one in ten patients which gave a broad picture of the level of care of the service as a whole. This example raises the issue of linkage between patient care cycles and clinical audit cycles, which are discussed in detail in Chapter 3.

Some therapists were involved in devising uni-professional goal attainment outcome scales by adapting existing scales for particular client groups. This is a challenging but intellectually complex and time-consuming task. Examples of this were efforts by speech and language therapists to adapt the Enderby scale (Enderby 1992) to different client groups. The scale had been designed for adults with head injury and needed to be adapted for other clients. A comment was that the scale was too general and that the one to five scoring system was not sensitive to small changes. With some clients, the scale is not suitable because the patient would never improve but, with good care, may remain in a stable state before a final deterioration. A group of therapists were devising a new scale that would measure change in the communication patterns of the patient's family and the frequency of distressing incidents.

We can see, then, that outcome evaluation remained, on the whole, at the level of patient care. However, we saw a few notable exceptions, usually not very developed, where work on audit outcomes was under way.

For example, a regional initiative to measure occupational therapy outcome for a small group of elderly patients was in progress. The patients were assessed on initial referral and at the end of the treatment period. The WHO classification of disability was used. It was planned that the final report would go to the regional health authority and the results would be fed back to therapists and communicated to purchasers. It was felt that, if positive, the findings would support the value of occupational therapy as a discipline.

In another example, the Canadian Occupational Performance Measure (Law *et al.* 1991) had been applied in three 10-bedded units and in a day care centre. The clients had complex mental health problems and challenging behaviour. Although broadly positive about the endeavour, the occupational therapists and nurses encountered problems in administering the scale because the patients did not cooperate. They were unused to being asked for their opinion.

A multi-professional mental health team in one centre was involved in a process of setting and reviewing goals. For each long-term patient, the team would set objectives over the next six months as well as longer-term aims. The six-month aims would usually be discussed with the patient. Sometimes the aim would be identified by the patient and agreed by the team as a way of improving the relationship between the patient and the professional. Expected outcomes (good and bad) would be recorded. The goals would be reviewed after six months and new goals set. The team had to make sure that they did not set goals that were too easy to achieve and to question continually the reasons for changing goals after six months (e.g. was it because the goal had been achieved and another was needed, or was it because the initial goal was the result of an incorrect assessment?).

The process of goal setting and measurement was educational and developmental for the team. They felt that from goal setting and assessment they would develop outcome standards that could be used in auditing the service.

In a physiotherapy service, the therapists were in the process of discussing how to improve goals by comparing groups of patients. If one group of patients had met all its goals and another had not they would discuss the reasons why and review the procedures and techniques used to see how to improve practice. This only entailed measuring individual outcomes of care but progress towards service outcome measures was planned. A comparison across client groups was already taking place and feedback was given to professionals in a non-threatening way.

Outcomes in mental health and learning disability

A problem presented to us was how therapists should set realistic common multi-professional goals for patients suffering from degenerative mental diseases. There is no real hope of improvement in health outcome and so the challenge is to set and measure goals related to the patient's quality of life. The same problem was identified for people with learning disabilities.

No clear distinction was made between process and outcome in the context of mental health rehabilitation. In the words of a clinical psychologist we met:

> If you are conceptualizing a problem as one that can be resolved or cured or got rid of, then the obvious outcome measure is whether or not you get rid of the problem and the acceptability of the resolution to the individual concerned. If one is talking about the context of long-term disability, whether that be physical or psychiatric, one is talking about the extent to which that disability handicaps the individual in their everyday life. One is not looking at whether or not you've got rid of the problem, but at the extent to which that person

is able to function and contribute with that disability. Those are actually two fundamentally different, both in physical medicine and in mental health, sets of outcome measures.

An example of a mature clinical audit activity that had completed one audit cycle and embarked on another is the individual care programme developed by Perkins *et al.* (1992). This audit successfully linked the patient care cycle to the clinical audit cycle and is described in Chapter 3.

Views on a multi-professional framework for audit

We now turn to the views we canvassed on multi-professional audit and the feasibility and desirability of a common framework for audit across the four professions and, more generally, their views on multi-professional clinical audit.

A common framework across the four professions

Views on the feasibility and desirability of a common framework across the four professions were mixed, but generally negative. A commonly held view was that there is no generic core across the four professions. Depending on the clients, different groups of professionals emerge that do not necessarily include the four together.

The client groups where the four professions worked together as a team included stroke rehabilitation, learning disabilities and, in some cases, mental health. With these client groups, it would be possible to envisage a common audit framework across the four professions, also including medicine and nursing, although there was the view that a national audit framework for each specialty rather than for the four professions together might be more useful.

A multi-professional framework

The organization of care delivery was felt to be of crucial importance to the development of multi-professional audit. Where professionals already work as a multi-professional team as, for example, in learning disabilities, the development of multi-professional audit was likely to be easier and would greatly benefit the patient. Multi-professional audit is therefore more likely to develop with some client groups than others, or when a multi-professional team collaborates on a specific clinical problem, for example swallowing difficulties.

One challenge to the success of multi-professional audit was to identify audit topics that were of interest to all parties involved. This is easier to achieve with client groups that require a multi-professional approach, such as mental health.

We met some therapists who regarded multi-professional audit as a threat, because it leads to de-skilling: 'as an OT, I want to stay an OT. I'm not trained to do anything else and sometimes if you amalgamate audit into a joint framework you might end up with a general mental health worker' (occupational therapist, mental health unit).

Similarly, multi-professional audit was perceived as a threat in the competitive atmosphere of some multi-professional teams where a perceived role overlap existed, such as in mental health. An important factor for the development of multi-professional audit is therefore an atmosphere of trust between professionals, a good understanding of each other's role and belief in the importance of the contribution of each profession involved.

Many therapists felt that multi-professional audit considers the effectiveness of a service as a whole, but not the effectiveness and input of a particular profession. They maintained that multi-professional audit should coexist with uni-professional audit. Multi-professional audit would be concerned with global measures and uni-professional audit with technical interventions specific to each profession.

There is the view that a common clinical audit framework is more likely to be concerned with process issues, and particularly the intervention of the team as a whole, rather than with outcomes. We note, however, that our findings do not support this view, since uni- and multi-professional audits were likely to be concerned with process in roughly equal proportions.

One solution mentioned is the coexistence of two – or more – audit frameworks that complement each other. A multi-professional audit framework measures the process of care of the team and its effectiveness; the uni-professional frameworks measure the process and outcome of specific technical interventions. This view was expressed by a clinical psychologist:

> Unless you've got a generic team of everybody being exactly the same, you inevitably need two frameworks. It's silly to try and make the same framework work for all professions because they are all a bit different. Having said that, a framework would be very useful because everybody's re-inventing the wheel in their own little way.

Elements of structure

In this final section we analyse the elements of structure that may affect clinical audit. We consider geographical, historical, organizational and status factors. We found no clear indication that history of a centre has an effect on the development of clinical audit. Other factors, however, we found to have some effect.

Diffusion

In principle, the geographical proximity of professional groups should be a factor affecting the propensity to joint or collaborative work or learning about clinical audit. Our research throws no clear light on this matter, but raises questions which remain relevant as the shapings or ecologies of health service organization change in response to the creation of trusts and, in the future, the abandonment of the regional level.

It might be assumed that those professional groups in close proximity in, say, an urban district would be likely to have strong connections with each other on the development of audit. We have indeed seen such examples but also, equally, examples to the contrary. At the same time, we note that the professions working within a diffuse district kept strong connections with each other. The reasons might be quite simple. Those working in small groups in relatively remote sites might be all the more concerned to keep strong contact with fellow professionals some distance away.

Organizational factors

In effect, the diffusion factor was seen to be less powerful than organizational factors. Where either a region or a district gave a strong lead in audit matters, usually backed by funding, connection between different groups was stronger. Where a directorate structure placed a chief professional in an advisory, as opposed to a managerial role, its ability to hold together different working groups within a trust became less certain although, at least in one case, strong professional bonds ensured that good work was developing.

Connection between professional groups within the same organization, whether it be region, district or trust, seems necessary and appropriate. Technical procedures take time and resources to develop, and testing across a wide range of clinical situations can only enhance the verification of their usefulness. This being so, as systems become reorganized, it becomes essential that managers and leading professionals take care to ensure that good connection between otherwise unviable audit groups are sustained or created.

Professional mix in sites

Again, it seems likely, and has been observed as well in a parallel evaluation of the total quality management pilot sites (Joss *et al.* 1994), that specialties vary in the ways in which their practitioners work with the different professions and, consequently, feel able to work with them on clinical audit. The more 'permeable' of the medical specialties seem to include psychiatry, child health and care of elderly people and, although our evidence is patchy, we noted that the professions did work collaboratively with psychiatrists on audit. This no doubt reflects the way in which clinical care is organized in these areas of clinical activity.

It follows from this supposition that work in community trusts is more likely to be cross-disciplinary, and stronger connections might exist between medical and other professionals than in acute trusts, because the nature of the work tends to demand a more explicit team approach.

Consumer influences

It could be assumed that different areas of clinical activity are influenced differentially by consumer groups and that this would affect the approach to quality assurance. Again, however, although in certain areas, notably child health and mental health, consumer groups were more evident and active, we perceived very little influence from such groups on the progress of clinical audit. However, those concerned with mental health and learning disabilities were seeking to incorporate the views of carers in clinical audit.

Institutional status: trust or district control

Where a district retained the provider as well as the purchaser role (a diminishing category), we found evidence that the district acting as purchaser was in a stronger position to help drive clinical audit development. Within such arrangements, different patterns could be found. In some, the purchaser within the district acted purely as such in relationship with provider units, working through a negotiative and communicative pattern of relationship; whereas in others a top-down managerial relationship was still evident. By contrast, the relationship between districts acting as purchasers and trusts was likely to be based upon a negotiation in which, however, the sanctions implicit in the power to make a contract will surely become as powerful as those belonging to managers. We had the distinct impression that purchasers were still learning their way in establishing the needs which they wished to have satisfied and striking a meaningful contract with providers who were often, and understandably, ahead of them in specifying appropriate modes of audit.

Conclusions and implications for the development of clinical audit

Multi-professionality

In their initial efforts to develop an audit culture it is not surprising that uni-professional audit has been dominant. The professions were enthusiastic about a move towards multi-professional audit, although not at the expense of uni-professional activity dealing with specific aspects of clinical care and treatment.

The therapists we met were enthusiastic about developing multi-professional audit as long as it runs alongside uni-professional audit. A common audit framework that includes only the four professions was not felt to be viable because various other combinations would emerge naturally depending on the client group and the individual case.

A multi-professional audit framework, flexible so that it can be adapted to specific client groups, seems to be a viable option. It could incorporate the results of uni-professional audits, or exist alongside such audits. Uni-professional audits would, therefore, be mainly concerned with the process of care and the effectiveness of specific professional interventions, particularly where care is not delivered by a multi-professional team.

Substantive focus

The characteristics of clinical audit as we find it from the literature and database searches, and the interviews we held with key informants, reveal that audit activities have focused mainly on structure, process and outcome issues; outcome measures were being developed or assessed by the professions.

We have classified the range of audit activity we found according to their clinical allegiance (core clinical, closely associated and less closely associated), their focus and their uni- or multi-professional status. We also describe the methods and types of data used for audit. The methods used are classified as case presentations, peer review, criteria-based audit, adverse events screening and sentinel events, and patient surveys. We give examples of audit activities in each category. By way of comparison, the most common methods of audit described in the report of the nursing and therapy audit programme (Department of Health 1994c) are:

- audit tools and models (e.g. the Donabedian framework and Monitor for nursing)
- outcome measures (e.g. the Barthel Index, Nottingham Health Profile)
- innovative care approaches (e.g. diagnostic-related care protocols, care maps, collaborative care planning, critical paths)
- core standards for professional practice
- comparison of practice and service against provider and purchaser quality standards and against Patient's Charter standards and accreditation schemes.

Outcome measures

Many outcome of care measures we came across focused on qualitative statements of therapeutic effects. Therapists set goals for individual patients as part of their routine care. The review of these goals was a form of uni-professional care outcome assessment.

Moving from uni-professional outcomes of care on an individual patient basis to multi-professional individual outcomes is feasible and we encountered several examples. However, few links existed between the various uni-professional outcome measures used.

Progression from individual outcome assessment to service outcome audit is complex and there are fewer examples where this had been achieved. The difficulty for uni- and multi-professional patient care is to move successfully from outcome measurement of individual patient care to clinical audit outcome measurement and back again, so that each type of outcome measurement feeds the other. In the few places where some work was under way on this, we note two tendencies: uni-professional outcome measurement tends to be highly technical and follows clinical specialties; and multi-professional outcome measurement addresses broader, quality of life issues and tends to involve the patient to a greater extent in goal setting and measurement.

This suggests that the two forms of outcome can, and probably should, coexist. Uni-professional outcome measures are necessary for assessing profession-specific technical practice. The results might be integrated into broader multi-professional outcome measures.

One problem is the amount of time and expertise needed to know where to find and how to select suitable outcome scales and, even more so, to devise new ones. A related problem is the lack of computerized databases suitable for outcome measurement. Service providers are in the best position to determine appropriate outcome measures for their client groups but they need effective and adequate technical support, in the form of information technology and support staff. This is one of the constraints we found to achieving successful audit (see Chapter 5 for a discussion of the constraints and benefits).

These factors can affect the style and dynamic of clinical audit, although it proved difficult to make a clear link between any one set of factors and the outcome in terms of clinical audit. Three organizational factors (organizational structure, focus and type of client group) did seem to have an effect, whereas the effect of others (history, geography, consumer influences) is less clear.

In this chapter, we have shown the range and type of audit activities investigated during fieldwork. Chapter 6 draws on these data and examines the connections between audit and management. First, though, we look in Chapter 5 at perceived benefits and constraints of audit.

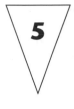

5 The benefits of and constraints on clinical audit

Sarah Robinson

In this chapter we discuss how far clinical audit has been shown to be beneficial or not in the improvement of clinical practice. In doing so we are modest in making judgements. As we have already noted, clinical audit has not got under way in any systematic fashion in all but a small minority of parts of the health service, and those implementing it have been too occupied in getting it started to attempt full evaluations of what they have been doing.

Moreover, participation in evaluation – and particularly evaluation where the results are open to colleague viewing – is antipathetical to traditional beliefs about professionalism, which take for granted both an altruistic regard for one's clients and individual competence to undertake specialist work without supervision.

In this chapter we again rely on what we could observe and record in our study of nine units in which clinical audit has been moving forward, with a view to both giving at least a conjectural account of the benefits perceived, and of ways in which others might contemplate evaluating their efforts.

The impacts of audit

The prime function of audit is to have a positive impact on the quality and effectiveness of care delivered to patients and clients, whether its focus is on clinical interventions or, as a secondary but important consideration, on the organization of the service within which these interventions take place.

It is thus of concern to ask what the impact of clinical audit is on the quality of care; what do those with professional, advisory and/or managerial responsibilities consider to be the value of audit; how far audit has an impact on their workload, sense of accountability, career prospects and morale, and whether it leads to an identification of training needs for themselves and their colleagues. Organizations installing audit will do well to take account of views on its value.

There is also the impact of audit on organizations both locally and nationally. Thus therapists were asked about its impact on their own profession. In our research, purchasers, provider unit managers (professional and general) and those with a district or regional remit for quality assurance were asked about the impact on resource management and contract specification, and on the relationship between the purchasing authority and the provider units. This organizational perspective on impact, like the individual perspective, is important to understanding the progress of audit, in that perceptions on whether it has a positive or negative impact on the profile of a profession and on resource management may well affect individual commitment to the enterprise.

Factors that facilitate or constrain progress

What were the resources and support relevant to audit and the incentives and disincentives to undertaking it? Several factors emerged that can either facilitate or constrain the progress of audit and the likelihood that it will have an impact. They fall into four main categories:

- availability of resources to undertake audit: these include time, finance and information technology
- audit expertise: this includes the experience and expertise of those involved in audit activities, and sources of advice to which they have access if needed
- aspects of inter- and intra-professional relationships: these include commitment to audit and perceptions of its worth, support for colleagues, concerns about confidentiality and potential impact of audit on particular spheres of work, and taking the lead in multi-professional initiatives;
- organizational issues: these include management structures, links between the various levels of an organization and between different organizations, and the ethos of sharing and of competition.

To demonstrate impacts achieved and factors affecting progress, we have selected for discussion two activities that varied in terms of type and complexity of form, level of maturity and range of health professionals involved.

Our detailed account of how these activities and their dimensions can be analysed is annexed to this chapter. The framework there deployed depends to some extent on our discussion of care and audit cycles in Chapter 3.

We now move on to more general findings in relation to first impact and then progress. These derive from our evidence of involvement in specific audit activities and from the broader context in which these activities took place.

Impact on care and service delivery

Almost without exception those whom we met said that audit had, or could have, a positive impact on the quality of patient care. Although they expressed this in a variety of ways, the essence remains the same. Audit provided them with the opportunity to assess their established practice and develop new ways of working to meet changing situations. This assessment provided the information necessary to identify deficits in provision and actions required for improvement.

An immense diversity of aspects of care and service provision were the focus of audit activities; some undertaken on a uni-professional basis, others involving two or more of the four professions, along with medical and nursing staff in some instances. The majority of these activities were at a relatively early stage of progress, and the number that had reached the later stages of the audit cycle concerned with implementing and monitoring change were fairly few. Those that had reached these stages had led to a variety of changes including:

- reduction or equalization of waiting time
- improved services for patients, such as refreshments and car parking facilities for out-patients, better maps to direct people to clinics, improved letters
- changes in discharge procedures, leading to fewer readmissions
- changes in procedures for record keeping, assessment and discharge forms
- equalization of workload between professionals
- development of new scales to assess progress and outcome in a range of client groups
- more effective appointment systems to reduce wastage of staff time
- implementation of procedures to ensure professionals keep in touch with long-term mentally ill patients
- introduction of short courses/training packages for staff, which focus on particular client groups or clinical problems
- obtaining new staff to remedy a shortfall
- introducing new posts in some areas, such as community link workers to facilitate discharge
- improved multi-professional communication and methods of working, in some instances through development of joint records, assessment forms etc.

The majority of activities we documented, however, were at earlier stages of the audit cycles discussed in Chapter 3. Standards setting seemed well advanced in all four professions as, to a somewhat lesser extent, did assessment of care against these predetermined standards. Equally frequently, the therapists described collation of information from patient and client records as a means of assessing achievement before moving on to devising standards. Many of the therapists involved in these activities (i.e. standards setting followed by assessment or vice versa) said that the exercise had a positive impact, whether or not action for change had as yet been identified. They felt that participation in these early stages of audit had increased their own professional confidence, enhanced their sense of accountability and improved the quality of care they provided. This was partly due, particularly in those activities entailing some kind of peer review, to learning from each other. While recognizing that improvement to patient care could not be demonstrated at this stage, they none the less felt that participation in audit itself leads to higher standards.

Impact on professionals

Although the focus of our investigation was impact on care, we explored the ways in which audit activities affected individuals; both positive and negative views were forthcoming. Involvement in an audit activity that had led to improvements in patient care, or had demonstrated that standards were being met, had for some been the source of pride: 'it was a real boost to our morale'. Involvement in audit activities was perceived as 'being good for the CV', and some therapists felt that it increased their chances of promotion. For example, 'I am recognized as someone with interest and experience in audit, this trust is very audit-conscious and so it could help if I applied to be the professional head of occupational therapy in the directorate.'

Another positive impact was the identification of educational needs of therapists; these included further training in the process of audit itself, and educational programmes on specific aspects of care or service delivery that audit had revealed as being deficient or requiring development to meet new situations.

But some, particularly more junior therapists, said audit had affected them adversely. Activities concerned with auditing record keeping were viewed as a means of 'checking up on them', rather than a way of improving patient care. Moreover, it was said to be an unfair method of assessment, because it did not acknowledge extremely heavy workloads. Other therapists feared that the impact of audit will be service reorganization that will reduce their autonomy and, in some cases, threaten their jobs. Some resented the paperwork generated by audit because it was often done at the expense of patient care. This view was particularly pronounced for staff whose involvement had been dictated by a senior professional, or who were involved in a multi-professional project led by a member of a profession other than their own.

Some of the heads of professional service commented that audit had a disheartening impact on staff because it made them realize how much more they could do for patients if they were not stretched to capacity.

Impact on professions and organizations

Impact on professions

A common theme is that audit activities were beneficial to the profession as a whole. Audit helped therapists identify their core skills and their contribution to care, and increased recognition of the profession by those in other disciplines. In the words of two heads of service: 'it has enhanced the standing of the physiotherapy profession locally, because we were the first to set up local standards, we're seen as the forerunner of standards work.' 'It has raised the profile of occupational therapy in the hospital, we now get invited to join all new projects.' And a therapist involved in a multi-professional project said, 'involvement has helped to demarginalize the profession in this trust.'

Many of those participating in multi-professional initiatives said that the involvement had increased their knowledge and understanding of the role of other health professionals. This led to a desire to develop roles in a complementary manner and to avoid duplication of effort. We heard also of multi-professional teams in which communication between different professions had been less than amicable. However, participation in audit meetings had provided the opportunity to thrash out difficulties and areas of overlap, resulting in a subsequent decrease of tension.

Impact on organizations

On the impact of audit on the concerns of those with general management or purchasing responsibilities, the evidence is somewhat contradictory. Within the same site, some managers said results of audit activities were used in resource management considerations, whereas others said that this was not the case. Similarly purchasers from the same health authority gave different accounts of the extent to which evidence of audit was included in contract specifications that involved services offered by the four professions. Therapists, however, were consistent in their views on this, in that they said evidence of audit was an important factor in securing contracts.

Perceptions of value

A less tangible topic centres on therapists' perceptions of what can be called the 'audit climate'. This concerns the way choices were made on aspects of care and service delivery to be audited, and whether therapists regarded these topics as relevant to their own professional concerns. It was this perception of relevance which seemed central to therapists' positive or negative views about the value of particular audit activities, whether driven by professionals or managers.

There were many instances of issues that professionals said had been of sufficient concern to motivate them into initiating audit of a uni-professional activity. There were also examples of multi-professional activities which had arisen out of the common concerns of those involved. However, the value of some audit activities was regarded with scepticism. For example, the number of clients seen within a given period of time and the time spent with each were common audit topics. Their value was questioned because the quality of the encounter should be the audit focus: 'guidance about audit produced by professional bodies at both national and local level is too concerned with time spent with each patient, rather than on the effectiveness of what was being done in the time.'

Examples of dissatisfaction with managers' activities include a management initiative following publication of the Patient's Charter: 'following from the Patient's Charter, my staff had to spend time on how long each patient waited – the paper work was enormous. It was pointless because we already had a system in which no one waited more than half an hour, so I said can we just record exceptions – but they didn't like this. Much of the paperwork is meaningless and it takes up staff time.'

Another aspect of concern about the choice of topics for audit was what some regarded as an overemphasis on outcomes. This entailed not only the exclusion of process but also excessive attention to those issues that could most readily be quantified. Topics for audit activities were chosen that would, it was felt, satisfy the managerial demand for outcome measurement. These were not necessarily topics which therapists felt were particularly urgent or important to the profession; they would, though, 'keep them off our backs'.

There is some evidence that, when asked to undertake audit activities for inclusion in contracts, therapists selected topics that they felt they could not subsequently be 'whipped by'; that is to say, they kept on safe ground rather than venture into more complex, although potentially more rewarding, areas of care provision and service delivery.

Factors that facilitate or constrain the progress of audit activities

We have noted that four main categories of factors emerged that can facilitate or constrain the progress of audit activities. Each is discussed in turn.

Resources

The resources available to undertake audit were regarded as inadequate. One therapist referred to the Normand team's recommendation – 'resources are needed if therapists are to undertake audit' (Normand *et al.* 1991a) – and went on to say that 'the necessary resources are still not available'. Discussions about resources focused on time, finance, and information technology.

Time
Lack of time to undertake audit was the major constraint on progress; the problem had two components. First, finding meeting times convenient for

all those involved in a particular audit activity was especially difficult for multi-professional initiatives, and was identified as one of the major constraints on the progress of multi-professional projects. Therapists who worked in the community said difficulties in finding mutually convenient meeting times for a multi-professional group were greater for them than for hospital-based staff: 'it's more difficult to get everyone together geographically, plus many community workers are part-timers and it's hard to find a time when everyone can get together. It shouldn't put us off, but it does.'

The second component was finding time to do audit. Very few said that they had been given a time allowance for audit activities; for most it was done in clinical time or in their own time. The heads of professional services recounted instances when their staff asked them if they wanted them to see patients or do audit, because they could not do both.

Lack of time for audit meetings and to carry out audit work had a number of effects. First, project schedules slipped and this became disheartening when an initiative had begun with a good deal of enthusiasm and commitment. Second, although a lot of audit activity was carried out in personal time because of individual commitment, this goodwill began to 'wear a bit thin' when nothing came of the work. Third, the lack of time acted as a disincentive to undertake audit in the future. Concern about lack of time was not confined to therapists; many provider unit managers admitted that finding time for audit was a problem for staff.

A variety of solutions were offered as to how this problem might be addressed, some of which had financial implications. Some therapists felt that the appointment of audit assistants to collect and collate data would greatly reduce the demands on their own time. Line managers were credited with telling staff that they could allocate clinical time to spend on audit. However, because no provision was made for the clinical work to be covered by someone else, therapists were faced with a choice of compromising care to patients in order to spend time on audit, or deciding not to compromise and therefore refusing to take part in audit. Nursing was contrasted favourably to the four therapy professions in relation to staff time, since bank nurses could be employed to cover nurses engaged in audit. At present bank systems do not exist in occupational therapy and, although some physiotherapy services do have them, they are not used to cover for staff who are involved in audit.

Finance
Views on finance varied. Some therapists thought the funds made available to regions by the Department of Health for therapy audit adequate, although most contrasted the amount unfavourably compared to medical audit. Some of the audits we came across were carried out entirely within existing resources, others were funded; amounts ranged from small sums for specific items to several thousand pounds. Many of the therapists in management positions said they could 'lose' the cost of audit for items

such as photocopying, stationery and secretarial resources in other budgets. However, when taking account of personal, unpaid time, the true cost of audit was rarely properly accounted.

Information technology

Information technology can make a valuable contribution to the progress of therapists' audit activities, including data capture systems for computerizing records and computer programs for analysing the data. Some therapists said that the systems they had access to were essential to their audit work.

Others had a number of concerns. First, many audits had been completed or were in progress without word processing or computerized data capture facilities; all the information was stored and analysed manually. This is an extremely time-consuming process and can be a disincentive to further audit activity. A second concern was the applicability of existing computer programs to the therapists' needs; some had spent time entering data on systems that had not subsequently been useful. Therapists emphasized the importance of being included at an early stage in discussions about the kinds of systems they needed.

A third concern was the accessibility of information stored in computers. We found several instances in which manual records were kept to back up the computerized records. In the words of one therapist:

> It's a new system, so there have been lots of hiccups and it's very slow to put things in. It's also a problem to get information out. When we kept manual records I could tell you at the end of every month how many patients, under which consultant, of which type we had treated and details of treatment. Now it's all in a computer which I can't access from here. The man in charge doesn't know what we want and what we want tends to evolve anyway. This database is the background for the project, as well as being used for records generally. But we have a backup of it all in notes and could extract it if the computer crashes.

There is no doubt that appropriate information technology systems would facilitate the progress of audit. Although some therapists did have access to such systems, others did not or had to use systems that were inappropriate or insufficiently accessible for their needs.

Audit expertise

Acquisition of knowledge and skills necessary to undertake audit depended on contact with therapists experienced in audit and easily accessed information and advice. Individual expertise was acquired from courses and workshops on audit and from learning from audit activities as one went along. Sources of information and advice were other therapists with audit experience, holders of quality assurance posts, published work and information networks on audit, and staff of specialist audit or research units.

Courses
Availability of courses on audit for therapists varied. One regional audit facilitator provided audit workshops at regular intervals; her approach had changed from waiting for groups of staff to ask her to do a workshop to setting up a series to which staff could sign up. Some therapists said they wanted more multi-professional events. A point made by some of the heads of professional services was that, although courses on audit were available, their continuing education budget was limited and staff chose to go on clinical courses rather than on audit courses when faced with a choice. This finding has been confirmed by studies of continuing education in nursing (e.g. Barriball *et al.* 1992) and in midwifery (Robinson 1994).

Experience and expertise
Therapists differed considerably in the amount of audit experience held; a few had been involved in audit for some considerable time, others were just starting out on their first project. Aspects they wanted help on were:

- writing a proposal in an appropriate format to make a bid for funds
- formulating specific objectives for the audit and not losing focus during its progress
- designing and testing data collection instruments
- methods of collating, analysing and interpreting results
- writing reports in an appropriate format to present to colleagues and those in a position to implement required changes in policy or practice.

Obtaining funding
Some therapists had received help in bidding for audit money from the region or provider unit; without this help they doubted whether they would have succeeded. One regional audit coordinator described the help she gave: 'I was able to . . . help them each write how they were going to take their projects forward and to put a costing against it . . . I rewrote little bits and got them into a pro forma that was acceptable and so all of these projects have now got their funds.'

Formulating and keeping to objectives
A difficulty encountered, particularly for multi-professional audit, was being able to specify the focus of the audit with sufficient precision to move forward into effective data collection and analysis. The audit activities we came across differed considerably in range and complexity of topic. An investigation into the association between waiting time after referral for osteoarthritis of the knee and subsequent outcome had a much narrower focus than one concerned with developing and auditing new referral procedures, new treatment protocols and new staff training packages for patients with dysphagia. However, deciding how process and/or outcomes could be assessed is a problem for any audit. Some therapists felt they had tried to cover too many outcomes or 'got bogged down with too much

data'. It was at this point that a discussion with someone more experienced helped to 'get them back on track'.

Clarity of objectives is important not only because it increases the likelihood that audits will be effective, but also because it helps maintain staff commitment. In the words of a therapist involved in a project which she felt was losing its focus, 'I'm in favour of the project but I'm not sure what are the next best steps with it and that's why I find it hard to find time for it.'

Designing data collection instruments

Measures used in clinical practice were often the source of data for audit even when the validity and reliability of process and outcome measures had not been confirmed. What therapists found a greater problem was how to design instruments for the specific purpose of audit: for example, a semi-structured interview to obtain patients' views, a questionnaire to staff on their training needs in relation to a specific aspect of care. Many needed advice and guidance. Others who had considerable experience of audit activities and instrument design were concerned about people's lack of awareness of the potential complexity of the enterprise. A doctor who had experience of medical audit and was now involved in multi-professional initiatives with a range of therapists said:

> My concern, when we were told about the excitement of multi-professional clinical audit, was almost the naïvety as to how simple it is to undertake audit, and I felt people were going to waste an enormous amount of effort and time drawing up half-baked, non-scientific research without realizing how difficult it is to construct good, simple medical audit to change things.'

Similar views were voiced by therapists with considerable experience. In the design of instruments, there is a close link between audit and research.

Some therapists did get help in instrument design and audit generally, usually from a quality assurance/audit coordinator post holder: The help was much appreciated: 'We've been very lucky to have . . . as a resource to use . . . we've been able to tap into her audit advice. We would have found it very difficult without her, to do any of the things we have.'

More often, though, therapists wanted guidance but did not know who or where to get it from:

> She [the audit facilitator] came and gave us advice – but I think we need much more guidance on instruments.

> At the moment, information about how to do it is patchy. We have had to make all our own contacts, we had to devise the questionnaire ourselves – there's been very little guidance.

> We've had very little advice on how to design forms and instruments. There probably is guidance, but it's not readily accessible.

Collating and analysing data, interpreting results and writing reports
Therapists also needed help with analysing and interpreting data. Those involved in large projects got bogged down with too much data and needed advice on how best to focus the analysis.

Getting the findings of an audit activity into an accessible form for dissemination was also difficult for those with little experience of report writing. Disseminating audit results is important if the outcome of the work needs discussion with other professionals or managers before changes can be implemented. Help at this stage by an experienced audit facilitator could ensure that the effort of undertaking the audit was not wasted.

The role of audit coordinators/facilitators
The work of audit facilitators consisted of providing courses and workshops about audit generally, encouraging staff to get started on audit, giving them advice during the audit process and, sometimes, taking over drafting the report for dissemination. Their help could be crucial to the success of an audit activity. These posts, though, were vulnerable; they might be the first to go in a cost-cutting exercise, or be left unfilled when holders became disillusioned with a series of short-term contracts and left. Therapists who lose this source of expertise may leave their audit uncompleted.

There is no doubt that expertise was building up but there were still many therapists struggling with audit without access to any kind of expertise. Those who felt that they were just beginning to develop some competence were often seen as experts by others; as one said, 'while we were doing the project, and finding out how to do it, suddenly our names were being given to loads of people, and we were being called in to advise them on their projects.'

Inter- and intra-professional relationships

Personal and professional relationships between staff, both within and between professions, had an impact on audit; some facilitated, others constrained progress.

Commitment and support
The heads of professional services we met were firmly committed to audit and devoted considerable time and energy to it. They said that, in the main, their staff were also committed to the principles of audit and supported their colleagues' participation in uni-professional and multi-professional audit activities. Some heads of service, however, found it hard to convince all staff of the value of audit, particularly when stretched to capacity with clinical work. Commitment occurred only if the results of audit were used; as one of them put it, 'junior staff who have joined audit activities become dispirited if it's not clear that the work is being used properly.'

Therapists involved in audit activities felt supported by their head of service and by their professional colleagues. This was the case for uni-professional or multi-professional audit, and when nursing and medical staff as well as members of other professions were included.

Personal conflict

The examples we came across were mostly of good interpersonal relationships conducive to successful audit, but instances of conflict that acted as a deterrent were given. This is illustrated by the following example, described by an audit coordinator:

> The two groups, community and acute, don't talk to each other. I've had one hell of a time getting them together to even talk about possible assessment tools that they might use ... I've chaired their audit meetings continually to try to keep them on a happy footing. If you've got conflict within the team anyway, trying to get them to question each others' practice is very difficult.

Confidentiality

Some therapists expressed concern about confidentiality in relation to other members of their multi-professional team and with regard to provider unit managers and purchasers. Audit that improves patient care depends on colleagues learning from each other and being willing to share results, both good and bad. This willingness to participate requires the proceedings to be confidential to those involved. However, with the move towards multi-professional audit, it might be more difficult to uphold confidentiality because of the greater number of people who would be involved. In one example, misunderstandings had arisen during a multi-professional audit because some of the participants felt that findings had been revealed to a wider group of people than originally agreed.

Another point concerned dissemination of information about audit activities and outcomes to managers. The pressure to do so has increased since purchasers have required audit information in service contracts. Some therapists regarded audit activities as the property of the profession to help them improve their service. Even though the guarantee of confidentiality should encourage a willingness to allow their performance to be scrutinized, some therapists feared that managers would use audit results to penalize staff.

A similar concern was the managerial demand for easily quantifiable outcomes. Therapists would choose topics for audit which were 'safe' and unlikely to lead to penalties. The result could be that serious issues of quality were not addressed.

Professional interests

Some staff were reluctant to participate in multi-professional audit because they feared it might lead to change in their practice or reduction in their autonomy in patient care. An example concerned an aspect of service delivery which most of the professionals involved felt was in urgent need of review. They could not proceed with an audit, however, because the professionals most likely to be affected by any recommended changes refused to participate. One of those involved said, 'it's so stupid because it's very personalized, as opposed to improving quality of care for patients ... it's sad because the service knows it has a problem but doesn't want to look at it.'

Implementing change

Reluctance on the part of some professionals to accept change recommended by an audit is a constraint upon progress, particularly, we found, when findings have an impact on medical staff. Conversely, supportive medical staff can make all the difference. They occupy a more powerful position within the organization and have greater influence on decisions to implement change than therapists. We have seen examples of both:

> With some consultants you feel as if you are talking to a brick wall, and that all the findings in the world you produce aren't going to make them change their practice, and they don't realize that this is going to have an effect on the rest of the team.

> You have to feel you are getting somewhere and that you are supported. I don't think we would have persevered with this if we hadn't had consultant support.

It is essential to discuss an audit activity from the outset with all those whom it might affect and to get their commitment. This is important even when the audit topic is peripheral to their work if changes planned affect their practice.

Taking the lead

An important decision in multi-professional audit is which profession should take the lead. We found that one or two key people naturally emerged. There was a tendency, though, for medical staff to assume, or be expected to take, the lead in multi-professional audit even when someone else was more appropriate. Therapists recognized that the medical profession has a much longer audit history than other professions, and they wanted doctors to share their expertise without dominating.

Organizational issues

Various aspects of the structure and ethos of organizations can support or inhibit the progress of audit.

Organization of professions

An issue of particular concern is loss of professional coherence when members are split across several clinical directorates. Lines of accountability for service delivery were to the managers of the directorate and not to the professional head of service. Therapists might work in directorates other than the one in which their head of service is based. Where this occurred the directorate structure could make it difficult to maintain strong professional leadership. This could reduce professional confidence, which in turn could undermine confidence to undertake audit, uni-professional or multi-professional. In the words of a therapist: 'multidisciplinary clinical audit will only be as good as uni-professional standards. People have to feel confident in their professional role and have to understand audit implications professionally, before they can go with confidence into multi-'.

Professional coherence was preserved when therapists formed their own consortium that provided services throughout the trust, rather than being split across directorates. Constant change in organizational structure within a trust inhibited the progress of audit. It requires time to devote to developing the new structures; time that might otherwise be audit time. Also reorganizations sometimes divide trusts into two, which impedes continuity of an audit project.

Links with management
As we have noted in Chapter 2, the extent to which heads of professional services had strong organizational links with managers at provider unit level varied considerably. In sites with strong links, managers could act swiftly in response to audit findings. A post for a community link occupational therapist, for example, was provided by management in response to an audit that showed deficiencies in the process of discharging patients home from hospital.

Where these links were weak, and managerial authority was required to implement the recommended change (e.g. if resources were required, or a change in service delivery was indicated), audit findings could get stuck because no structure existed through which to channel them. There can also be a lack of interest by managers in the findings, particularly when these relate to care delivery over a long time-span, as is the case for clients with learning disabilities or continuing mental health problems.

Sharing information
Mechanisms for sharing information about audit activities were important to achieve progress. The opportunity to learn from each other's mistakes lessened the likelihood of 're-inventing the wheel'. Informal networks were often generated by quality assurance advisers who put people in touch with others working on similar audit topics, and directed people to sources of written information. Informal mechanisms of this kind, however, depended on particular individuals; if they left, then a long time might have elapsed before a replacement was found, or the post might have been left unfilled. Formal audit networks were less common. Attempts were made to enter details of audits into computerized databases but, as we noted earlier, not all therapists had access to a computer. Reports on audit

activities were often found at trust and region level but did not reach staff engaged in audit.

The separation of purchaser from provider inevitably risks loss of clear channels for disseminating information about audit. Professional networks were more clearly defined and used for dissemination than organizational networks.

Some therapists were deterred from sharing information about audit beyond the provider unit. The managers took the view that findings from audits are business secrets and not to be divulged. If information about audit is to be used as part of the process of bidding for contracts from purchasing authorities, then providers will be reluctant to share information with competitors if the likelihood of securing a contract is jeopardized. This was more of a problem for organizational audit, however, than for audit of clinical practice. One therapist said: 'we always check out with people how much they are willing to share. If I'm issuing information about anything, whether to purchasers or to other trusts, I always check with the chief executive or director of operations and say I want to talk about this . . .' And another: 'Some trusts are now banning sharing information about audit, because it's business secrets. This government has said you are in competition.'

Just at the time when involvement in multi-professional clinical audit is becoming more widespread among health professionals, as a result of the policy from the NHS Executive, the competition of the internal market may serve as a deterrent to establishing a common body of audit knowledge and expertise.

Undertaking audit: implications for the future

Can we conclude that the factors noted in this chapter will lead to a successful or unsuccessful clinical audit outcome? Although certain factors did help or impede progress, we cannot impute a direct causal relationship. For example, some audit activities were well resourced in terms of facilities and expertise, but failed to make an impact because of poor links with management, or because resource priorities prevented an action being implemented. Other audits did not make progress because of time constraints, lack of clerical support and inadequate advice on how best to proceed. We have noted some audit activities that made a positive impact without resources; they succeeded through the motivation and commitment of energetic therapists. Others that had resources did, of course, succeed too.

None the less, clear messages emerge about factors that facilitated audit and those that hindered its progress. We can comment on those elements to which attention should be focused if audit activities are to develop effectively.

There are two issues to consider in relation to the development of multi-professional rather than uni-professional audit: is it desirable and is it feasible?

Some professionals thought all audit should be multi-professional, but most said that aspects of their professional practice, particularly their therapeutic work, should be audited on a uni-professional basis. Multi-professional audit is ideal for assessing the overall strategy of a service, however. We found examples of where such a strategy was lacking because commitment to audit and provision of resources in one part of the organization were not matched in others. It makes no sense, for example, to make a time allowance for audit if there is no mechanism for transforming outcomes into practice, or in providing funds for clerical assistance but no access to expertise in instrument design.

Taken as a whole, our findings indicate that a coherent strategy should contain the following elements:

- resource and educational provision
- commitment to audit at all levels of health service organization
- clarification of the audit agenda
- recognition and support of the role of key people.

Resources and educational provision to enable people to undertake audit were therapists' main concerns. Lack of time, perhaps more than any other issue, was seen as a constraint to progress. How time is allocated and to whom needed to be considered, also the cost of audit. While many audit activities had been greatly facilitated by Department of Health audit money, much of the work was uncosted (such as time) or funded from other budgets (e.g. clerical assistance, photocopying). Some therapists had access to appropriate information technology systems; others did not. Moreover, the time it may take for them to become familiar with computer programs needs to be recognized.

The importance of and need for adequate educational provision and access to expertise were frequently voiced concerns. Therapists wanted guidance on all aspects of the audit cycle, from formulation of aims through to monitoring impact of changes. But help with designing data collection instruments and interpreting results was wanted the most. It is essential that assessment is made at the outset of an audit project, by someone with experience, on the expertise required throughout its course; and then the expertise must be acquired. The provision of training and access to sources of advice and information was patchy. It is unrealistic to expect people without research training to design valid and reliable instruments; they should have access to research expertise in the organization or in nearby institutions of further or higher education.

Commitment to audit, at all levels of health service organization is an important component of an overall strategy. We have seen many instances of lack of interest in audit findings by general managers or lack of channels, beyond the professional head of service, for disseminating findings. Ensuring that mechanisms exist for translating findings into action is essential if commitment to audit by therapists is to continue. This means

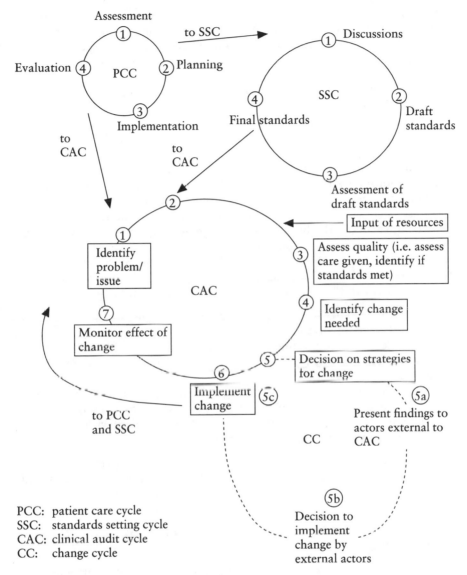

Figure 5.1 Possible connections between the various cycles

thinking through all possible ramifications of the seven stages shown in
Figure 5.1 (described with examples in the annex to this chapter).

Closely related to commitment is the perception by different groups of
the audit agenda. Health professionals were concerned that their motivation to improve quality of care had suffered under a cost-cutting managerial agenda. While no one disputes that delivering high quality care as

efficiently as possible should be the aim of the service, this should not be done at the expense of quality. Moreover, by focusing on cost and efficiency, the more complex, and probably more important, aspects of care are not audited. If commitment to audit is to be maintained, people need to be clear about its purpose and convinced of its value.

The centrality of key post holders is crucial if audit initiatives are to continue successfully. Heads of professional service and holders of quality assurance posts are such key people. They need continuity and stability of employment, and support, if they are to support staff undertaking audit, and disseminate findings. The structure of the organizations in which they work must permit them formal and regular access to those with a managerial responsibility for health care policy and resource management.

Audit activities at varying stages were widespread among the four professions. There was a great deal of commitment, many audits were successfully completed and the body of knowledge and expertise was expanding. Audit was undoubtedly responsible for some positive impacts on the delivery of care and on the education and careers of therapists. At the same time there is evidence that a coherent strategy for audit was lacking. The main problems in this regard can be summarized as follows:

- insufficient resources and expertise available to therapists involved or expected to be involved in audit
- varying levels of commitment to audit and a failure for initiatives to come to fruition when professional and/or managerial commitment is lacking
- different perceptions of the audit agenda, and a degree of uncertainty and in some cases cynicism about the purpose of the exercise
- weakness in the organizational position of post holders with a key role in initiating and sustaining audit activities.

All these issues need addressing if commitment is to be sustained and if the time, money and effort that is invested is to be worthwhile. Models and guidelines as to how this might proceed are the subject of Chapter 7.

Annex: procedure for evaluating the impact of clinical audit

Here we describe a procedure that can be used for analysing audit activities. We go on to apply the procedure to two audit activities that we have seen. One succeeded in moving through all stages of the clinical audit cycle; the other had not got that far. This exercise may help practitioners and managers in their audit endeavours.

We found that the reality experienced by professionals was more complex than that postulated in our cycles framework in Chapter 3, so we developed the cycles in a bit more detail. For example, 'implement change' is Stage 5 in the original clinical audit cycle (Figure 3.1), but becomes Stage 6 in the clinical audit cycle, of Figure 7.2 in Chapter 7 because an intermediate stage emerged ('decision on strategies for change'). The development of the interrelationships between the cycles is also depicted in Figure 7.2; for ease of referral, we reproduce it here as Figure 5.1. First we describe the analysis procedure developed from the cycles framework. Then we present, as examples, two audit activities to show their impact and the factors that supported or constrained their progress round the clinical audit cycle.

The analysis procedure developed from the cycles framework

In this annex we are concerned with the progress made with audit activities and so we focus on the clinical audit cycle and the change cycle depicted in Figure 5.1. By conceiving these two cycles as a sequence of seven stages, we can visualize how audit might proceed and with what impact.

Stage 1: identify aim of or problem for audit

The first step is to specify the aims of the audit activity or define the problem to be investigated. Is its focus the structure, process or outcome of care, or a combination of two or all three? Some activities have a single aim based on a known problem, e.g. reducing length of time between a GP referral and hospital appointment. Others have many aims: for example, to assess existing information available for stroke patients, devise new packages of information, and then evaluate their impact.

Stage 2: set standards

The second stage is to set the standard to be reached for the audit activity. This might require movement into a separate standards setting cycle, as depicted in Figure 5.1, or the standard might be agreed without difficulty, e.g. the time between GP referral and the hospital appointment will be no longer than one month.

At this stage it is wise to consider the resources available to enable the audit to take place and have an impact. Resources include funds, time allowance, information technology, expertise and managerial support.

Stage 3: assess quality (i.e. assess care given and identify if standards are met)

This stage involves assessing or measuring the quality of care and establishing whether the standards have been met. Outcome measures that can be used are described in Chapter 1 and some of the methods we have witnessed are discussed in Chapter 4. The extent to which this process can be facilitated or constrained has been noted in Chapter 5.

Stage 4: identify change needed

The fourth stage of the cycle entails identifying whether action or change is needed and, if so, what it should be and how it might be implemented.

Stage 5, 5a, 5b, 5c: decide on strategy to implement the change
A series of decision-making procedures is probably necessary before the change needed can be translated into action. Who makes these decisions will depend on the focus of the activity, the types of changes needed and whether they have resource implications. That is to say, it might be appropriate to make the decisions within the clinical audit cycle or outside it. The progress made at this stage is crucial for determining whether an audit activity has an impact on the delivery and organization of care.

5: decision making within the clinical audit cycle   Practitioners may be in a position to decide what change is needed and to go ahead and implement the change without recourse to managers or other professionals. This is most likely with an audit of a technical aspect of care relevant to one profession solely and so would be a part of the clinical audit cycle.

5a and 5b: decision making by people outside the clinical audit cycle   Other audits have implications for people – other professionals or managers – outside the clinical audit cycle who would share in, or take over, the decision making. Changes identified in the course of a multi-professional audit, for example, would be negotiated with members of all the professions involved. Some audits identify changes that require managerial input, either because it involves a change in policy or because additional resources are required, or both. Achieving an impact thus depends on passing on the findings of the audit to relevant members of other professions and to the appropriate level of managerial decision maker (Stage 5a of Figure 5.1) and obtaining agreement for the proposed changes and resources (Stage 5b).

Stage 6: implement change
It is at Stage 6 of the clinical audit cycle, which coincides with Stage 5c of the change cycle, that an impact is made on the way in which practitioners give care or how it is organized. As shown in Figure 5.1, this stage feeds back into either the patient care cycle, in that aspects of care may be changed, or into the standards setting cycle, in that new standards may be devised or existing ones revised.

Stage 7: monitor the effects of change
The final stage of the clinical audit cycle entails monitoring the effects of the change; that is, 'closing the loop'. This can be the start of a continuing improvement process and so Stage 7 would become Stage 3 of a second audit cycle, or rather, spiral.

The impact of audit activities and the factors that affected their progress

We move on now to describe two audit activities as examples. Each is considered in terms of Figure 5.1: how far round the audit cycle it went, what impacts were generated on the way, and what factors facilitated or constrained progress.

Activity 1

Topic: Equity of access to physiotherapy services.
Level of maturity: Stage 7 of the audit cycle: monitoring effect of change.
Professionals involved: Physiotherapists and general practitioners.
Source of information: Interviews with senior physiotherapist and audit facilitator, and written documentation.

Progress of Activity 1 round the audit cycle

Stage 1: identify aim of or problem for audit The aim of the activity was to achieve, on a trust-wide basis, an equal waiting time for physiotherapy services for GP-referred patients. The initiative came from senior physiotherapists concerned about considerable variation in waiting time from one physiotherapy services site to another.

Stage 2: set standards No specific standard was set other than that the waiting time for all patients would be equal. The physiotherapists did not feel able to set a definite time-scale at this stage.

As regards input of resources, clerical resources were made available 18 months after the audit started.

Stage 3: assess quality The method used was to ask GPs to refer all patients needing physiotherapy to one site which could be used as a clearing house, rather than to several as previously. The physiotherapists at each site were asked to contact the senior physiotherapist at the clearing house site once a week with their current waiting list. Then new referrals were allocated to the site nearest the client's home, or to the site nearest home with the shortest waiting list.

Stage 4: identify change needed The process described in Stage 3 revealed that there was a three-month waiting list for physiotherapy services. Previously some clients had been seen sooner, whereas others had waited much longer. Two actions for change were identified: the policy of referral to one centre and subsequent allocation should continue so that access would be equitable; and an increase in the physiotherapy establishment was needed to reduce what the professionals regarded as too long a waiting time.

The senior physiotherapist wrote a report on the findings and on the changes indicated.

Stage 5: decide on strategy to implement the change   As shown in Figure 5.1, this stage can have three elements:

5   the physiotherapists agreed to pursue a policy of equal access and to follow the clearing house policy
5a the case put by the physiotherapists to the general practitioners per-suaded the GPs to pursue the policy of equal access
    request for resources: the GPs agreed to put a request to provider unit managers to fund another physiotherapist
5b the unit managers agreed that there was a need for this and would check their budgets for the necessary funds.

Stage 6: implement change   The agreed actions specified under Stages 5 and 5a were implemented but the unit managers were not able to release the funds for another physiotherapist (5b).

Stage 7: monitor effect of change   Equity of access was monitored on a continuing basis by the senior physiotherapist. Equalization of waiting times was achieved across the trust but the waiting time remained at three months.

Factors facilitating and constraining Activity 1

Resources   No time allowance was made for the physiotherapy staff in-volved in this project; the work involved was done in their own time or in clinical time. Clerical resources were made available 18 months into the project; before this the physiotherapy staff dealt with their own secretarial and record-keeping tasks.

Education/expertise   The regional audit facilitator gave advice on how to carry out the audit and how to collate the results.

Inter/intra professional support   According to the senior physiotherapist most of the physiotherapists and general practitioners were very support-ive. A few GPs were initially resistant because they thought the central clearing house idea would slow down the process of referral; but once they saw that the policy worked they supported it.

Impacts of Activity 1
This audit had an impact on the nature of service provision in that waiting times were equalized across the trust. It also demonstrated to the physio-therapists that they can influence management decisions, in that an in-crease in staff was agreed (although did not materialize). The staff saw the benefit of audit and became less hostile to it. Little by way of resources (either time or money) had been forthcoming, yet the activity had suc-ceeded in being driven round the audit cycle by the determination and

enthusiasm of the superintendent physiotherapist and her senior colleagues to improve the service they offered patients.

Activity 2

Topic:	Improving information provided for stroke patients and their carers at home.
Level of maturity:	Stage 3: assessing quality.
Professionals involved:	Occupational therapists, physiotherapists, social worker, nursing and medical staff.
Source of information:	Interviews with head of occupational therapy, senior community occupational therapist, senior physiotherapist, social worker, clinical director and general manager

Progress of Activity 2 round the audit cycle

Stage 1: identify aim of or problem for audit   The general manager wanted a multi-professional audit initiative and called a meeting of all health professionals to decide on appropriate topics of common concern. Two were selected, one of which was to improve quality of information provided to stroke patients and their carers. Selection of this topic reflected professional concerns about what, in their view, was the negative and unnecessarily alarmist nature of much of the information available. The focus was thus to improve the process of giving care and the outcomes achieved in terms of patient knowledge.

Stage 2: set standards   Setting specific standards was premature for this information-gathering exercise but the protocol for the audit identified the following short-term aims:

• to assess appropriateness of existing information
• to find out what information patients have, how helpful they found it, and what else they would like to know
• to put together an information pack based on outcomes of the first two aims
• to document information given to patients in hospital in their records.

Long-term aims were to monitor patients' reactions to the new information pack, and to set up support groups in the community for stroke patients and their carers.

Regarding input of resources, no additional resources were provided; work had to be undertaken within existing budgets and workloads.

Stage 3: assess quality   The professionals met to plan and discuss progress once a month; so far they had met twice. The intention was to meet more frequently in future and also for sub-groups to meet on specific aspects of the work entailed. They had decided to assess the appropriateness of exist-ing information by reviewing videos available for stroke patients, and had made a start on this. They also agreed to obtain information from patients by means of a semi-structured interview schedule; this was to be admin-istered to patients in hospital and also after their discharge so that they could convey any needs for information that they felt unable to express when in hospital. An interview schedule was designed.

This was the stage the audit had reached when we met it. A small num-ber of patients in both settings had been interviewed to test the schedule.

Factors facilitating and constraining Activity 2

Resources   All the therapists identified *time* as the major constraint to the progress of this audit. It was extremely difficult to find times when they were all able to meet and work together; the coordinator said that this was a particular problem for multi-professional audit work. Also, the thera-pists were under pressure to find time for the tasks required by the project, given their clinical case load. As one said, 'I haven't got the time to do it and I feel I have to give patient care priority over this audit project. It's harder to give time to things that are long term.' The audit coordinator said that she needed consecutive time to get the audit really moving, per-haps a month; trying to squeeze it in around other demands prevented continuity of thought and progress.

Regarding *finance*, a bid had been made for £500 of regional audit money. Everything needed (cost of the videos and photocopying) had so far been found within existing resources. No secretarial resources were available and so group members did their own typing.

There was no access to *information technology* for a computerized record system and so all the record keeping had to be undertaken manually.

Expertise, experience, education and commitment   All the staff were en-thusiastic about the audit's potential for improving the quality of care. They enjoyed working on it and were committed to its progress. By the second meeting they felt they had begun to 'gel as a group'. Only one member had previous experience of audit; they all said they needed more training. Expert advice had been available at the first meeting from the regional audit coordinator, who had helped with formulating aims and deciding on the most appropriate way to obtain and evaluate the informa-tion required.

A major problem was lack of guidance on designing and evaluating the interview schedule. One member was concerned that data obtained in the pilot study contradicted her clinical experience and she attributed this to the schedule's design. No one knew where to get guidance.

Inter-professional and management support   In the main the staff felt supported by other professionals who were not directly involved, and by the general manager, whose initiative had led to them embarking on the audit.

Impacts of Activity 2

The audit cycle had not been completed but already one impact was that the therapists had more knowledge of the role of the other members of the health care team involved in the care of stroke patients. They all hoped that providing accurate and relevant information to stroke patients and their carers would enable the staff to both lessen patients' distress and empower them to ask the right questions at the right time. It should also help to make their own work more effective: they spent a lot of time undoing the harm done when patients were given inaccurate information. Provision of accurate information at the outset would give them more time for other aspects of the rehabilitation process.

Conclusion

This annex has demonstrated how audit activities can be analysed for their progress and stage reached in the clinical audit cycle. We have described the kinds of impact that emerged from specific audit activities and the ways in which progress was facilitated or constrained. The procedure could be used by practitioners and service managers to assess progress made in their own audit activities.

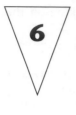

6 | Clinical audit and managing health systems

Tim Packwood and Anémone Kober

How is clinical audit used by health service managers? We begin by differentiating levels of management and the nature of their concerns with audit, for the professional service managers, the general managers in the provider units and the purchasers. We then illustrate the form of audit leadership and identify some of the principal features of managerial involvement. We next consider the particular perceptions of audit held at the different management levels previously identified. Next, the implications of the management role are considered. Does a considerable degree of managerial involvement give clinical audit a particular character? Does it bring particular strengths and weaknesses? The chapter concludes by typifying some features of the managerial connection. As in other chapters, evidence from our research is used to illustrate and illuminate the argument throughout.

Management and managerial concerns with audit

Managers and management play a considerable part in clinical audit. This is hardly surprising: stronger management in the service has been an objective of government policy over the last two decades (Flynn 1992; Harrison *et al.* 1992) and increased managerial involvement was an element in the moves to formalize audit across the service following the NHS Review (Secretaries of State for Health 1989).

Although management is performed by individuals, it has collective purposes. Hoyle (1981) defined it as a 'continuous process through which members of an organisation seek to coordinate their activities and utilise their resources in order to fulfil the various tasks of the organisation as efficiently as possible'.

So, concentrating on the managerial role in audit means looking at the organization in a particular way. The focus is on the working relationships that integrate the work of disparate individuals, on the allocation and control of resources and the achievement of organizational goals and objectives, rather than on, say, the technical aspects of the service provided to patients. It is a feature of the four professional disciplines which are the subject of this book that, while they undoubtedly possess accepted professional properties, such as expertise, considerable autonomy in their work and external professional bodies to define desirable standards, they work within hierarchies with an appointed senior manager who is accountable for delivering a service to an accountable standard. Such a professional service manager can instruct other staff from the same profession and shape their work. In clinical psychology, however, which is closer to medicine in its organizational arrangements than the other three professions, the extent of the managerial relationship *vis-à-vis* other qualified staff is more ambiguous. The professional service manager will be a qualified and experienced member of the relevant profession, although time to practise professionally is likely to be limited.

Until the introduction of general management, the four professions were usually functionally organized and managed in health authority district-wide services, managed by members of their own profession and clinically autonomous.

Since the introduction of directly managed units/trusts, different organizational models have emerged, including management in one unit/trust with services contracted to others, or services divided between units/trusts and managed within each.

This largely has resulted in the demise of district level posts, although a few became advisory with management responsibility for one trust and an advisory function across several others. Simultaneously, allocation to care group/medical specialty directorates occurred, or amalgamation in 'support' service directorates under general management by professionals (or non-NHS professionals).

A common model is one in which accountability goes through a professional service manager, to a unit general manager, although accountability may be divided between management and professional advisers/leaders. Some trusts have established directorates composed entirely of therapy services or have included them as part of clinical support services.

In all of the six major sites which we studied, senior professional service managers were accountable to higher level general managers within the same unit, although in one case, because the structural revisions following the NHS Review were still to be made final, accountability remained shared between general managers in the provider units and district-based heads of the individual therapy services. Where the provider unit is organized on the basis of its major service functions (in a hospital this is the directorate or department, in the community this is the care group or patients' service), accountability may be to the relevant director or care group manager. This was the case in two of the six sites, but in four cases accountability was broader, to unit-wide coordinators, such as directors of supporting or operational services. In one case accountability for one of the therapy services remained direct to the chief executive of the unit. As noted earlier, therapy services staff might also find themselves under dual management: accountable professionally to their own professional service manager, and operationally, in respect of their day to day work, to a general manager running a locality service or a service centre.

Whatever the case, and organizational arrangements appear to be in constant flux, general managers, who may be drawn from any NHS discipline or from outside the service, are in a position to impose requirements on the various professions. Within the internal market, their influence will, in part, stem from contracts that the provider unit has agreed with purchasers, and purchasers' requirements therefore represent yet a further influence on clinical audit. Indeed their influence is to be strengthened under the revised arrangements for audit, which suggest allocating audit monies to lead purchasers who are required to negotiate contracts for clinical audit with their provider units (Department of Health 1994b). The existence of different priorities between purchasers and providers is explictly recognized in the 'model contract'.

The different sets of managers delineated above have different interests in audit and use it for different purposes; and these interests and purposes are different again from those of the professional practitioners delivering services to patients:

- professional service managers are concerned with the management of a service, integrating the activities of the practitioners to best effect and providing, allocating and controlling the necessary resources
- general managers have a broader concern, integrating the various services provided by the sub-unit (directorate, care group) or unit as a whole
- purchasers are concerned to obtain 'value for money' care for their population of patients. This relates back to
- service practitioners, who are concerned with the quality of care they can deliver to patients.

These different perspectives of audit and quality assurance were categorized in a recent evaluation of total quality management (Joss et al. 1994) referred to earlier, where three modes of quality assurance were distinguished:

- *technical*, concerned with the specialist quality of processes of care, applied by individual providers in their work
- *generic*, concerned with the common aspects of quality in the way that work is organized and managed, its results and relationships, as applied by whole services or management units
- *systemic*, concerned with the quality of a comprehensive and integrated set of services to meet the health needs of a local population, as applied by a trust or required by a purchaser.

Table 6.1 Different perspectives of audit

	Concern	*Mode of quality assurance*
Professional service managers	The individual service	Technical, generic
General managers	Services provided by the sub-unit or unit	Generic, systemic
Purchasers	Services available to the local population	Systemic, technical, generic
Service practitioners	Services given to individual patients	Technical

This categorization can be applied to the framework of managerial interests developed above to sharpen the perception of different managerial perspectives and purposes (Table 6.1).

The assumptions underlying these categorizations are first, that from a managerial perspective clinical audit needs to be multifunctional. Second, if it is to satisfy various managerial purposes, and be used to its full potential, it has to draw in a wider set of actors than the professional practitioners and include general managers and purchasers. The extent to which clinical audit was able to secure involvement at different levels of management will be discussed at the conclusion to this chapter.

But taking for the moment managerial interests in audit as a whole, the importance of managerial involvement can present itself in two ways: first, in the considerable number of audits that are undertaken to satisfy managerial accountability. This can be seen not just in the general sense that managers are charged with making sure that audit happens but also in the specific nature of the topics audited. From a managerial perspective audit emphasizes the management of services, their inputs, the control of their processes and their outputs, rather than focusing on the nature of the technical processes applied. Almost the complete opposite emphasis is found if clinical audit is compared with the early development of medical audit (Packwood *et al.* 1994). A great deal of what clinical audit encompasses is, in fact, auditing the organization of services. Second, since therapy practitioners are employed within a management hierarchy, managerial authority and commitment are likely to be central in making use of audit and achieving change.

Managerial influence and involvement within audit activities

In our research for each audit activity investigated we assessed whether it was led by the professional service manager, by another manager, by the therapists collectively, or a combination of actors. In order to carry out this classification, several factors were considered:

- who initiates (or requests) the audit activity?
- who carries out the work involved?
- who monitors the activity progress?
- what reporting mechanisms are used? (reports, informal discussions etc.)
- what are the lines of accountability for audit?
- who uses the results of the audit, and for what purposes (does it mainly inform managerial decisions or not?).

Several actors were identified as leading and directing audits:

- professional service managers
- therapists (individually or in a group) and multi-professional care teams
- general managers (including service managers)
- medical consultants
- purchasers (however, only one purchaser was directly involved in driving audit, so this category was amalgamated with that of general managers).

In some cases, an audit activity belongs to more than one category. For instance, an activity initiated by a professional service manager but carried out by a group of therapists who determined its priorities belongs to two categories 'professional service managers' and 'therapists'.

Table 6.2 shows who were the main actors leading audit and whether the audit activities were uni- or multi-professional. Professional service management provided the main or shared drive for a majority of audit activities (94). By contrast, general managers provided the drive for 19 activities, as did teams and individual therapists; medical consultants led 6 audit activities.

Managerial interest within clinical audit and the character of managerial audit

The uni-professional nature of professional audit

Nearly all the audit activities driven by professional management were uni-professional in nature (76 against 18). This is not wholly surprising as all the professional service managers were heading a uni-professional service.

The reverse is true for the activities driven by other actors. Thus, 7 audit activities initiated and driven by teams of therapists or individual therapists were uni-professional but 12 were multi-professional. The general managers were the driving force behind 13 multi-professional audit activities, and 6 uni-professional ones. The 6 audit activities led by medical consultants were multi-professional (and of course they were brought to our attention because they involved other professions).

The pattern that emerged is one where uni-professional clinical audit is driven by professional concerns, whereas multi-professional audit is more likely to be driven by a variety of actors: general managers in the provider

Table 6.2 Leadership of the audit activities by type of audit (uni- or multi-professional)

Type	Leadership of the audit activities			
	Professional service managers*	Therapists'teams*	General managers (including 1 purchaser case)*	Medical consultants*	Other
Uni-professional	76	7	6	–	–
Multi-professional	18	12	13	6	1
Total	94	19	19	6	1

* Audit activities in these sections can belong to more than one category

and purchasing units, teams of therapists, medical consultants as well as service heads.

Focus of audit

Table 6.3 presents the leadership of the audit activities investigated according to their focus (structure, process, outcome) and their category (core clinical audit activities, closely associated activities, less closely associated activities), as defined in Chapter 4. It must be noted that these categories are not mutually exclusive; an audit activity can address structure, process and outcome issues at the same time. It could be expected that managerial audit would emphasize structure and process, and less closely associated audit activities.

A majority of audit activities driven by professional service heads, alone or in combination with other actors, were linked to process (76). Approximately equal numbers addressed issues related to structure and outcome (38 and 43 respectively).

The professional service heads were slightly more likely to initiate and/ or lead activities related to closely associated activities (46), than core clinical activities (37) and less closely associated activities (35). Professional service heads were particularly involved with audits linked to processes of care and closely associated activities. They occupy the interface between technical and generic concerns.

Projects initiated wholly or partly by teams and/or individual therapists were more likely to be linked to process (16) and outcome (16) than structure (7). This seems logical, considering the greater clinical involvement of therapists. Similarly, teams and/or individual professionals appeared slightly more likely to be involved in core clinical audit activities (10) than closely associated audit activities or less closely associated audit activities (7 each).

General managers were more likely to have initiated and/or driven audit activities linked to structure (13) and process (12) than outcome (9). On the whole, general managers are likely to be more interested and competent in generic and systemic matters rather than technical.

Although linked to process, the nature and topics of most audit activities were managerially orientated. Topics were often related to caseload management (e.g. waiting lists, Körner data, computerization of caseload). These audits clearly addressed generic purposes and could contribute to systemic concerns if the results are used to inform general managers.

Another type of audit activity often initiated by service heads at departmental level is educational and developmental in its focus. This was especially apparent in clinical psychology. In some sites, regular case presentation meetings were held at departmental level and were organized by the professional service head. These initiatives tended to be uni-professional and took place within a managerial structure. They were initiated and monitored by the professional service heads but they addressed core technical issues.

Table 6.3 Leadership of the audit activities by focus and category

	Professional service managers	Professionals/teams	General managers (including 1 purchaser)	Medical consultants	Other
Structure	38	7	13	2	1
Process	76	16	12	4	–
Outcome	43	16	9	2	–
CA 1	37	10	9	3	–
CA 2	46	7	1	4	–
CA 3	35	7	11	2	1
Other	–	2	1	–	–

Audit activities in all sections can belong to more than one category

CA 1: core clinical audit activities
CA 2: closely associated audit activities
CA 3: less closely associated audit activities

Definition and analysis of different managerial interests

Professional service management

The role of professional service managers
Managers are known by a variety of titles depending on the local organizational structure of the unit/trust. We came across professional managers with titles such as, for example, head clinical psychologist, acting head speech and language therapist, manager of the occupational therapy services, director of physiotherapy. This points to the diversity of organizational structures encountered during fieldwork.

In most sites, professional heads were also service managers. However, in one site, their professional responsibilities were separated from day-to-day managerial responsibilities, which were delegated to locality managers in the community trust.

The professional service managers were highly influential as initiators, leaders and also as actors who were often in a position to bring about change. Their functions in relation to the audit activities were varied:

• they acted as initiators
• they kept the momentum of audit going and were often the ones making sure that audit was kept on the agenda at departmental and other meetings
• they took decisions in relation to the audit projects
• they passed information to their own line managers, thus acting as links between the professional and the general management structure
• they were either actively involved in most stages of the project or were kept regularly informed
• they used the data/results from the audit process in order to inform their own managerial decisions. Frequently the results were communicated in the form of reports and/or discussed at meetings with general management
• in some cases the results informed the contracting process.

The professional service managers had often been involved for quite a few years in quality assurance activities. Standards setting was an area where they had been active, starting as a uni-professional activity at district level, and involving professional heads of discipline.

Personality is important. In districts with proactive professional heads, audit developed early (late 1980s, early 1990s). In one site, audit had developed in the late 1980s as a result of a combination of the initiative of senior managers in the unit and in the service itself. In another site, the development of multi-professional clinical audit was partly the result of a proactive head of department who had initiated links with the local medical audit committee.

Lines of accountability
The line of accountability for audit usually follows the managerial lines. Professionals report to their principal, chief or superintendent, who in

turn reports to the professional service manager. The professional service manager reports to a general manager (e.g. director, care group manager), not to a director of quality. Audit is usually one element identified and discussed during individual performance reviews/annual staff appraisal schemes.

The lines of accountability for multi-professional clinical audit are much less likely to follow the professional lines than is the case for uni-professional audit. Either there were no formal lines of accountability, or there were informal lines of accountability to the leader of the audit, who was often a medical consultant.

In the site where the professional heads only had an advisory role, audit lines of accountability also followed the managerial lines, which meant that above superintendent level, accountability was usually to general managers.

When such persons exist, audit coordinators are identified by professional managers and professionals as useful intermediaries. They do not belong to the managerial structure and are perceived by professionals as 'less threatening' than professional or general managers. As outsiders, they can 'step back'. However, the lack of managerial clout of these coordinators means that they have little power to request participation from professionals in audit activities.

In one site, the professionals identified dual lines of accountability for audit: either following the managerial lines, via senior professional staff, or via the audit coordinator. The audit coordinator was accountable to the professional service manager.

In most sites, responsibility for audit was usually vested in a few people: the professional service manager and the senior or middle professional managers accountable to her/him. This model follows professional lines, 'the [head of service] would be the initiator [of audit] given that a large part of the audit systems in the department are actually done in the super-visory relationships' (clinical psychologist, head of rehabilitation).

Below the middle management level, delegation of authority for audit is often difficult. In one site, there was a clear lack of commitment and enthusiasm for audit below the level of chief speech and language thera-pist. This situation may have been due to the therapists' large clinical workload. Another factor was that the therapists felt that the topics cho-sen by the professional managers were not relevant to clinical practice. Audit, coming down the management line, was felt to be an imposed chore.

Use made of audit results
Decisions to implement change are mainly effected by professional service managers, although professionals are usually consulted and kept informed at staff meetings. When the change was important, the professional man-ager often needed to consult his/her own line manager. It was noted in a few sites that decisions taken by professional managers within their sphere

of authority got acted upon whereas when decisions needed to be referred to general management, no action was taken. This suggests that the clinical audit cycle includes the change process when the change identified falls within the sphere of authority of the professional service manager. Inversely, when the change identified lies outside of the sphere of authority of the professional service manager, the process of change moves into a separate, but connected, change cycle (see Figure 5.1 in Chapter 5). In many such cases, the professional service managers then act as the link between the clinical audit cycle effected by professionals and the managerial change cycle, effected by general managers.

One of the main uses of audit data by professional service managers is internal monitoring of their service. In one site, the caseload of each clinical psychologist was computerized and monitored regularly. In another, waiting lists were audited for each specialty clinic of the service. This enabled the professional service manager to take action in order to reduce the longer waiting lists.

One way that professional management enforces change is to point out to the professionals the weaknesses and needs of the service as identified by the audit. This process of making the professionals aware of the need for change is a subtle way to put pressure on them to redress any omissions or weaknesses in their practice or delivery of the service. One example related to caseload monitoring. Circulation of data showing the imbalance of caseload and waiting lists in different clinics encouraged the professionals with lighter workloads to offer to help others. This was then referred up the professional management line for approval. This process of helping out across clinics was possible because the budget was held by the professional service manager, who could readily make the necessary adjustments. However, this was likely to change as the budget would in future be held by a general manager for the whole of the care group.

In at least one case, audit results were discussed at team meetings, targets for change identified, and the results monitored internally by the team on a regular basis.

Professional service managers at the interface between general management and professional services
As we have noted, professional service managers are usually accountable for audit to their own line manager, usually a general manager. This often takes the form of sending audit reports at regular intervals (often yearly, in some cases quarterly).

In at least two sites, however, general managers were pressing service managers towards multi-professional audit. Usually, general managers were more interested in multi-professional audit than uni-professional audit and more likely to request it.

In some cases, there is a supra-departmental audit and quality council or committee. Membership of these committees includes professional service managers, medical directors and general managers. The focus is very much managerial. Success and degree of influence of these committees is variable, but generally low. In one site, there was a quality council for the unit whose terms of reference were to develop and monitor clinical audit initiatives, but it was felt to be a 'toothless' committee.

There was at least one example of a unit-wide, largely top-down audit activity. This involved implementing and monitoring a care programme approach in a mental health unit. The implementation of the programme was the responsibility of the multi-professional teams. The audit was carried out by a monitoring group that included mainly professional service managers and general managers. This monitoring group itself was a subgroup of a working group that included, among others, senior managers from the provider unit and professional service managers. The standards which were monitored were related to managerial concerns: national requirements such as the Patient's Charter and local requirements set by purchasers. The reporting mechanism was through annual report to the unit general manager. Appropriate feedback had not been given to the teams and this was felt to be a problem that needed to be rectified. Some respondents felt that this top-down approach from senior management was not the best. Autonomy from senior management and enthusiasm for audit at team level were felt to be interdependent.

It must be noted, however, that a commitment to audit from senior management and a supportive environment are often cited as essential ingredients in promoting enthusiasm among professionals. Conversely, professional service managers appreciate their freedom in setting the agenda but feel a need for strong support for clinical audit from senior managerial staff, both in the provider and in the purchasing units.

In most sites, the services could follow their own agenda on audit, especially when they were proactive and ahead of the requirements of the purchasers. It was often felt that this would change once purchasers and general managers became more knowledgeable about clinical audit.

At the time of fieldwork, clinical audit was often an activity controlled by professional service managers but detached from the wider managerial framework. There is a need for strong and good connections between professionals, professional service management and general management.

Relationships with purchasers
Purchasers were in general not in a position to influence specific audit projects. However, in one site, the district quality office audited the services and directly influenced the choice and nature of audit topics by making prescriptive recommendations. And in two other sites the district had an explicit expectation that the providing units would undertake audit activities.

The types of audits that professional service managers led were linked in some cases to purchasers' requirements or areas of concern. These requirements were usually included in the contracts. They were often related to national guidelines (e.g. the Patient's Charter) that had been translated into the local contracts. One principal speech and language therapist said (with reference to the Code of Practice developed in respect of the 1991 Education Act), '[t]here is a legal requirement to provide advice within six weeks and we find that we are not able to do that. So I set up a process to identify why the system was breaking down.'

The areas that had to be monitored according to the contracts with purchasers included face-to-face contacts with patients (Körner data), waiting lists and waiting times. These areas were often the ones where professional service managers had initiated audit projects. Professional service managers were thus aware of purchaser's requests and took them on board. Some felt that there was a lack of interest on the part of purchasers for clinical audit. This lack of encouragement and recognition for work done demoralizes therapists.

In most sites, professional service managers had led purchasers in relation to clinical audit. The general feeling was that clinical audit was well ahead of purchasers' requirements. However, these requirements were likely to intensify with the introduction of service-based agreements. Clinical audit was still fairly autonomous, but this was likely to change.

Different types of relationships with purchasers existed:

• in one site, there was a lack of contact with the purchasers and the managers in the provider unit. 'Audit started from the professionals, is uni-professional and was assisted by national professional initiatives. There is no lead from the purchasing unit or local medical initiatives or from local management' (professional service manager)
• in most sites, there was some contact with purchasers through the contracting process. Clinical audit was not, however, requested in the contracts. Monitoring of activity data was usually requested and professional service managers complied
• in two sites, the relationship with the purchasers was closer, and involved negotiations and audit training of purchasers by some professional service managers
• finally, in one site, the district health authority quality office carried out an external audit of all the units. Topics for internal audit and improvement were identified after these visits. This prescriptive, top-down approach creates a feeling of insecurity among some therapists and generally gives external audit a bad name.

The importance of audit for career development
Many professional service managers thought that audit improved their career opportunities. Some felt it provided them with useful managerial knowledge: 'Audit is very important for careers that might not just be clinical but managerial too. It's understanding really about management, budget and funding' (chief speech and language therapist). Audit experience was felt to be particularly useful by professionals who were already engaged in a managerial career and wished to pursue this road.

General management within provider units

In our interviews with occupants of general management roles, respondents ranged from chief executives to heads of particular care groups, patient services, or of community health care centres at the sub-unit level.

There are clear perceptions that general managers, whether carrying unit-wide responsibilities or exercising responsibility for services to a particular clientele, are becoming more aware of clinical audit and feel a responsibility for ensuring that it is taking place. Audit responsibilities have become written into their contracts of employment and, in some cases, the responsibility has been sharpened by the need to produce an annual audit report and, latterly, an audit plan. In part this is a by-product of the need to exercise control over the organization and, in particular, to monitor the adherence to contracts. Quality initiatives provide a means to this end and clinical audit is one among a number of tools that come to hand. Ways in which clinical audit was mentioned as potentially serving as a managerial monitoring tool were as a means of determining priorities, and as a component that contributed to the maintenance of a business plan.

As an element in unit management, clinical audit can contribute to policy making and planning, although respondents did not believe that it had played a significant role to date: 'clinical audit is not yet informing the agenda at the macro level' (general manager for elderly/physically disabled services).

But clinical audit was also regarded as a quality initiative *per se*, to be used 'for their own improvement' (associate general manager, medical directorate). The problem here is that it proves difficult for managers to know how far any improvements stem from clinical audit, as against other quality initiatives or indeed from other managerial activities.

If general managers are going to be able to use clinical audit, they need to be able to influence its content. There were only a few examples where this had occurred, but general managers felt that if the need arose they could require professional service managers to include particular topics within the remit of clinical audit. One example presented was of a manager requiring a therapy service to obtain patients' views as part of its audit activities.

But if managerial involvement is acknowledged to be a good thing, it is clear that it was starting from a low base. Hitherto clinical audit had not been a major priority for general managers. Three reasons could be discerned:

- general managers had been, and to an extent still were, heavily preoccupied with implementing the structural changes that stemmed from the 1989 Review
- as mentioned above, it proved difficult for managers to untangle clinical audit from all the other quality initiatives. From a management perspective they are all bound up with getting value for money from service

inputs and are largely seen in terms of the general standards contained in the Patient's Charter (Department of Health 1991a) and Health of the Nation (Department of Health 1991b), which were being introduced across units and sub-units. At the operational management level, audit is seen as part of the customer-focused culture, concerned with patient satisfaction rather than the technical objectives set up by the clinical teams. General managers had little appreciation of the technical standards required to review process in clinical audit. And there was appreciation of a danger, as expressed by a care group general manager, 'that the current emphasis on evaluation produces superficial quality, only concerned with those activities that can readily be audited'.

- adequate data for clinical audit are not always available. Managers accepted that the therapy services required access to activity and financial data if they were to review their management of care, but generally they lacked the capacity to supply what was required. The resource management initiative had not yet been rolled out to all the provider units in our sample and nowhere had it reached the point where the professions could use it as an aid to audit.

So mainly general managers had left the development of clinical audit to the professional service managers: 'audit is not, therefore, linked to the management of operations. It is essentially a means of peer review which has considerable importance within the professions primarily concerned with treatment' (director of operations).

There was some feeling that, more than representing a pragmatic response to circumstances, managerial distance recognized an issue of principle: the professions needed to gain a sense of 'owning' their audits and external management involvement would be counterproductive. 'It would not be the ethos for the directors to shape the agenda of clinical audit' (director of operations).

The practitioners might interpret managerial involvement in audit as interfering with their staffing and work processes, which would act as a disincentive. Further, managerial involvement would be likely to prove redundant. Some general managers see provider services as relating directly to purchasers on quality issues without requiring a managerial intermediary. The purchasers are likely to be increasingly prominent in shaping the audit agenda.

The problem with devolving the development of clinical audit to the therapy professions is that managers see them as developing the process at different rates and in different ways. If clinical audit does mean multi-professional audit then such disparities present problems. At one level the uni-professional approach is commendable because it means that the different professions are developing audit systems which they 'own', but managers want audit systems in place in those services which include many professions. The ideal might be a mixed system: multi-professional audit of a common core of issues, with uni-professional audit of specific professional issues.

Although not overly involved with clinical audit to date, the general managers did suggest a number of encouraging auguries for their future involvement. First, medical audit is, by government decree, to become translated into clinical audit. Management has gained some experience of working with, and making use of, medical audit and this experience will spill over to the clinical audit undertaken by the professions. There will also be increased resources available to support the therapy professions in their audit initiatives. Locality managers and managers of service centres already have experience of promoting multi-professional audit. Second, the 'contract culture' of the NHS is likely to spread within provider units, and therapy services/directorates will have to market their services to other directorates through service agreements. These quasi-contracts, which will be overseen by general managers within the provider units, might well include a clinical audit component. And, finally, there are welcome signs that audit is beginning to shift its focus from inputs and process towards outcomes. This will increase its utility.

Purchasers

As yet, purchasers do not appear explicitly involved with clinical audit. They clearly have an implicit involvement through their concern that services should meet required standards and levels of quality, but these are general in their nature. Purchasers will define care standards that apply across the board in all of their contracts and add in specific standards for individual services. The standards and levels are also heavily reactive to central government concerns. They mirror the Patient's Charter and Health of the Nation and emphasize the control of service inputs.

A further reason suggested for the lack of direct influence is that purchasers' concerns, particularly as far as community services are concerned, are with patients' services, such as learning disability or care of the elderly, not with the services provided by individual disciplines. So purchasers require a multi-professional approach to the maintenance of standards and quality, whereas to date clinical audit has basically been a uni-professional activity. Clinical in this sense has meant non-medical audit. These responses from purchasers confirm views expressed by general managers in the provider units, and by the professional service managers in therapy services. The purchasers' concern is with quantity of services rather than with quality: 'the professions are more advanced as regards quality. The purchasers are not using this professional knowledge' (chief executive). And perhaps as a result, it is exercised, vicariously, by the providers themselves.

A good example of this latter tendency is provided by the service specification set for one of the professions by the major purchasing authority at one of our sites. The service specification required that 'quality standards will be set for all aspects of care within the departments and will be kept under continual review by quality assurance checks and clinical audit.' Further, 'all staff will be appropriately qualified and experienced, and will conform to professional standards and the code of ethics as set by the respective professional bodies.' The planning and delivery of the service was required to 'take account of local issues and regional and national guidelines'. The service was then required to audit itself each year by applying five procedures from the following list of possibilities:

- special interest groups (peer review)
- individual performance review (IPR)/clinical appraisal (CA)
- identification of training requirements from IPR or CA
- staff meetings with a regular agenda item of quality assurance and with minutes and actions
- monitoring of complaints and plaudits
- consumer satisfaction surveys
- monitoring workload levels, waiting lists and waiting times
- case rate review
- monitoring re-referrals
- identifying unmet clinical service demands
- providing an annual report to the purchasing authority.

The above list was applied to all the four professions but provision was made for the inclusion of specific requirements for individual professions.

The absence of direct involvement with audit was not wholly a matter for regret. There was a view that it was right that purchasers should not be too involved in how audits were undertaken, what was audited and what was not; they should merely satisfy themselves that audit was being undertaken. This is, first, because the content of audit was seen as a professional, educative matter, 'a way in which they [the professionals] can reassure themselves about the effect of their work' (director of public health). Audit was seen to be different in this respect to other quality initiatives, which were a matter for purchasers as well as for the managers of provider services.

Another director of public health took this professional view of audit further, defining it from a medical perspective as 'scientifically assessing some aspect of clinical care', a way of ensuring that the results of clinical research can actually work in practice. A further reason for leaving the detail of audit to the service providers was to encourage the latter to feel that they 'owned' their activities, and had discretion as to how they should be developed. This would be impossible if audit were to be dictated in any detail by the purchasers. This argument accepts that it may be beneficial if the results of audit feed into service contracts but the process is bottom up. The results of the providers' formative evaluation of their own activities are fed to the purchasers as part of contract negotiations.

But the viewpoint described above, essentially justifying the *status quo*, was challenged by a rather more proactive vision of audit: 'The more we know about what services are being provided, and the views of the clients, the more that we can be satisfied that we are buying what our residents would need. So we would obviously encourage clinical audit as much as possible' (director of public health).

With this approach, clinical audit will become less of a do-it-yourself activity by the providers, as purchasers become increasingly involved with the process. They have a variety of different means at their disposal:

* annual reports, including annual reports of audit activities
* meetings with the providers, where audit topics and their results can be discussed
* service reviews, which can include a review of audit and what it has accomplished
* informal networks, linking purchasers and providers, which could give the former indications as to the application of the audit process.

Such strategies could be readily adapted to the conditions of the audit process. Reports on audit activity, for example, could be structured to match the framework of the audit cycle, reporting on standards set, processes reviewed and changes implemented. An emphasis could be placed upon auditing outcomes of care rather than its management. The approach would be formative and might indeed bring purchasers and the service providers together, as was perceived to be the case by general managers: 'Contracts confirm what is agreed, they do not create it' (director of health care standards). And audit requirements can always be explicitly set out in a contract, although this would be moving towards a more summative view of audit, a move which the majority of respondents would appear to regret. In the words of a quality manager working for a purchasing agency:

> Clinical audit from the purchaser's point of view is a tool to the purchaser to know that standards set within the profession have been delivered, yea or nay, and if nay, were the standards inappropriate or what are the training implications, what needs to be changed? It's not going to be too long before purchasers are going to want clinical audit to be auditing outcomes and effectiveness of care and services, so that we know that what we purchase has a proven benefit.

Characteristics of managerial involvement in clinical audit

Clearly audit strongly reflects managerial interests. The nature and topics of most audit projects were managerially orientated. This managerial orientation appears, at the time of writing, to owe more to the involvement of professional service managers than to that of our other two categories: general managers and purchasers. This may, however, be changing. Indeed the involvement of professional service managers appears to be a crucial factor in the success of audit activities. They are able to employ their authority and professional status to initiate and progress audits and to utilize their results, often in the face of some reluctance from practitioners with other calls upon their time. Pollitt has suggested a spectrum of possible

1 Give general exhortation to develop a quality assurance programme, but no incentives or sanctions
2 Offer positive incentives to develop a quality assurance programme, but no sanctions
3 Require professionals to develop a quality assurance programme, with penalties for not doing so
4 Require professionals to develop a quality assurance programme and specify key features of the system
5 Require professionals to develop a quality assurance programme and specify key features of the system and directly participate in the system
6 Require professionals to develop a quality assurance programme and specify key features of the system and directly participate in the system and claim right to use disaggregated data.

Figure 6.1 Six quality assurance approaches for managers in a professionally delivered service
(From Pollitt 1990)

approaches for managers in relation to quality assurance (Pollitt 1990), as depicted in Figure 6.1. Professional service managers appear to occupy the interventionist end of his scale: requiring the professionals to participate, specifying key features of the system (and in many cases initiating the system), directly participating in audit activities and using the data produced. Use is partly associated with their own professional practice but also with their managerial roles which they draw on in reaching judgements as to how the service, and individuals within it, are performing. This gives clinical audit a decidedly summative feel.

A further feature of this reliance upon service managers is that it may push audit in a particular direction and emphasize particular characteristics. Professional service managers occupy an important organizational interface between professional and managerial concerns for the operation of their services. They are concerned with both the process of individual patient care, and therefore with the technical mode of quality assurance, and with structure and outcomes, and therefore with more generic concerns for the quality of the service as a whole. Both these concerns are likely to mean that they emphasize uni-professional, as opposed to multi-professional audit. It is also the case that some activities, that were classed by some professional service managers as clinical audit, might be more accurately described as management. Staff appraisal is a case in point. It could be argued that the dominant managerial influence of the professional service managers brings significant advantages and disadvantages: advantages, in that service providers enjoy a degree of freedom in shaping their own audit activities, and that strong uni-professional audits, capable of impacting on individual care cycles, can occur. It also brings disadvantages, in that the ability of professional service managers to link services audits with wider organizational and comprehensive patient service developments appears weak. Strong multi-professional audit is also weakened, both because it relies upon initiatives from general managers, and in some cases doctors, which are not always forthcoming, and because it lacks the clear focus of responsibility provided for uni-professional audit by the professional service manager.

Our evidence also suggests that the presence of an audit coordinator or facilitator is valuable for promoting audit within a particular professional service because he or she can mediate between professional and managerial concerns.

However our study also suggests the existence of a kind of watershed for the involvement in audit of both general managers and purchasers. So far they have, for a variety of practical reasons and principles, been largely reactive to the service providers as far as audit is concerned. It was widely perceived that this state of affairs was likely to change. Purchasers must now include the undertaking of audit within their contractual guidelines. Within the new arrangements for clinical audit, their role is becoming more important, taking the lead in determining priorities, and this is likely to extend to GP purchasers. Purchasers were already seen to be relating directly to the service providers on audit issues. The new government policy and advice regarding the development of clinical audit would also require a stronger input from general management. In terms of Pollitt's categorizations, the approach of both purchasers and providers is moving from the non-interventionist, giving general exhortation for clinical audit, to requiring professionals to engage in clinical audit and, in some cases, going further and specifying key features of the system and requiring access to aggregated data.

Analysing managerial involvement

One popularly held view of clinical audit is of a bottom-up activity, driven by the concerns of the professional peer group to improve their quality of patient care. On our evidence there is some truth in this perception. Service providers have been perceived as taking the lead in the development of clinical audit and this interpretation would account for the importance of the technical mode of quality assurance.

However our evidence also suggests that this model would need to be modified in at least two respects: the driving force is the professional service managers, rather than the providers themselves; and there is a gulf between professional service managers and general management, a gulf which makes it difficult for the technical mode to pass up the structure and contribute to wider generic and systemic quality concerns.

An alternative view of clinical audit, and one perhaps looking more to the near future, is of a top-down activity. Audit was activated in a professional managerial structure which was, in theory, set within a larger organizational framework: 'this cascade model would ultimately be set within the contract negotiated between the purchaser and the provider unit' (clinical psychologist head of section).

This model treats clinical audit as any other quality strategy, to be implemented through the managerial hierarchy. Thus the strong influence exerted by professional service managers vis-à-vis service providers in audit activities is to be expected, and, indeed, encouraged. It is also appropriate for the results of audit to be used by managers in a summative way, holding professionals to account.

However this model would also require qualification in that there is little evidence as yet of much audit activity cascading from top to bottom of the structure. There is also a particular gap with reference to the involvement of general management within provider units, although this may be strengthened in the future as directors of quality come to play a stronger role in coordinating and integrating all quality assurance initiatives, providing a source of advice to general managers on audit matters. There is certainly some evidence from our research of purchasers relating directly to service providers and their managers to promote the technical and generic aspects of quality assurance for their patients.

Our evidence suggests that both models have something to offer: the bottom-up emphasizes technical process and focuses on the management of a service, promoting strong uni-professional audit; and the top-down emphasizes the generic quality of service provided by a unit or sub-unit, and the systemic quality required by a population or sub-population, promoting multi-professional audit.

For either model to be developed to the maximum would appear to require two elements: first, general management needs to be more engaged in the audit process, to provide a generic view of quality and link this into the wider systemic vision; in particular, general managers would need to be involved with each step of the clinical audit cycle, so that the process of identifying the change needed, and of implementing it, remains part of the cycle. Second, mechanisms at different organizational levels need to bring the different managerial interests in clinical audit together. These might comprise:

- at the service providers/professional service managers' interface we found that specific audit meetings were relatively rare, although audit was commonly taken as an item at staff meetings
- at the professional service managers/general managers' interface audit/ quality committees were common at the unit level, although professional service managers from the professions would not necessarily attend. Formal audit meetings at the sub-unit level (the directorate or patient services group) appeared rare, what interaction there was typically taking place on a one-to-one basis between a professional service manager and the relevant general manager. According to the NHS Executive, provider organizations 'will need to develop clinical audit plans at both organisation and clinical team/directorate level' (Department of

Health 1994b), so there is a strong case for providing appropriate mechanisms

- at the interface between general management in the provider units and the purchasers, government policy requires purchasers and providers to negotiate priorities for audit and for the lead professional(s) for clinical audit from the provider unit to be involved in contract negotiations with the host purchaser and participate in the contract review process. The creation of a formal audit or quality committee linking the two interests would provide a forum for negotiation and review and would, incidentally, be perpetuating an organizational arrangement that had been found helpful by some participants in the early days of medical audit (Kerrison *et al.* 1993)
- if the purchasers wish to get to grips directly with the quality of service provision, they may wish to relate directly to the service providers on audit matters, rather than relating at second-hand through the reporting mechanism or through general managers. As noted earlier, we found some evidence that this was the case from our research. Purchasers' review of service contracts could be used to negotiate audit issues and monitor subsequent action, although there would be a question as to whether purchasers possessed the necessary expertise to negotiate issues largely concerned with technical process. Undoubtedly, too, some service providers would experience too close a relationship as interference.

A final point concerns the accountability for clinical audit. Professional service managers combine in their persons both professional and managerial accountability, potentially producing strong uni-professional audit. It may be that the development of multi-professional audit requires strong general management direction, from a point in the structure above the professional service manager. Although some multi-professional audits have developed from the situation of different professionals working together on patient care, these initiatives do seem to have difficulties in locating the accountability for progressing the audit process and the authority to act upon any results.

Although different types of manager will wish to use audit for different purposes and in different ways, this chapter has drawn attention to the importance of involving all managers, at all levels of the service, with the audit process and with the application of its results. But, for once, the message is not disputed; an imminent upsurge of managerial interest in audit is being widely predicted by the therapists we met. The next and final chapter suggests how this interest might effectively be applied, through formalizing clinical audit as a crucial part of an operational quality-promotion system.

7 | Making audit a workable system

Maurice Kogan, Sally Redfern and Anémone Kober

The starting point for change

Clinical audit is firmly on the policy makers', managers' and professional practitioners' agenda but, in many ways, has hardly begun to form a useful and practicable course of action in a health service which is undergoing such large-scale change. It has not been comprehensively developed as a multi-professional activity. The trusts as we saw them in our research were not yet bridging the gap between different forms of medical and clinical audit. There were no formal links between nursing audit and clinical audit, or clinical audit and any other form of quality assurance. In most sites, audit remained internalized to the individual professions. Knowledge from clinical audit was not being used for generic care purposes or for resource allocation. Clinical audit was not contributing much to the wider organizational setting.

At the same time it was clear that many committed and knowledgeable professionals were building up audit systems and competence and that in time medical audit would merge into multi-professional clinical audit.

We are thus at a formative time when the health care professions should take the opportunity to secure ownership of clinical audit. At the same time managers can consider how best to use the knowledge generated by audit to improve their knowledge of the activities for which they are accountable.

From all of our work with professionals, we are certain that deliberate and thought-through plans of action, drawing on wide multi-level and professional support, are a necessary prerequisite of audit. This will make audit more competent in terms of its technical content and usefulness to professionals. At the same time, the demands of both accountability and of purchasers' contracts mean that the development of audit cannot be tackled haphazardly and without regard to the wider organizational picture.

In this final chapter we bring together points made earlier which should enable health care managers, both general and clinical, to begin the task of building their own audit arrangements and procedures. We offer here propositions from which they might make choices about the form and content of audit. They concern:

- the purposes and content of audit
- the ways of mandating it, and the mechanisms through which it may be achieved
- the knowledge generated by audit
- the ways of evaluating the effects of audit.

In order to make use of some of the explanations offered earlier in the book for application to policy and practice we repeat some key tables and figures from previous chapters in what follows.

Some ways forward: components of modelling

How might the professions begin to model their arrangements for clinical audit? The main decisions on content of audit they should make are:

- identify the main components of audit, as illustrated in the cycles in Figures 7.1 and 7.2, and select those relevant to their specialization(s). In particular, professionals need to determine clear and relevant clinical audit topics
- discuss the audit project with all those on whom it might have an impact (including patients and general managers) in order to ensure their support for change
- at the outset of the audit, assess the type of expertise needed to carry it out and make links with the appropriate sources
- determine the sequence of audit procedures: whether they are to be in a reiterative cycle or in spiral sequence, or some other logical pattern
- determine the connections to be made between the patient care cycle (or other type of sequence) and the audit sequence
- ensure that proper connections exist between the different cycles; in particular, that findings from clinical audit are transformed into action (connection between the clinical audit cycle and the change cycle) and are fed back to the patient care cycle
- establish, in collaboration with both professional and general managers, the extent to which audit is likely to, or should contribute to, generic or systemic audit or other forms of quality assurance
- determine the substantive focus of the audit: that is to say, outcomes or process analysis. In this context, an outcome measure can consist of a series of interim outcomes from different processes.

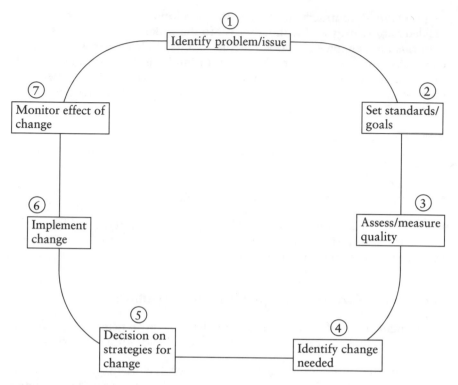

Figure 7.1   The clinical audit cycle

What should audit contain?

Although the cycles are presented as containing essential elements in particular sequences, which are sometimes found to exist in practice, they are no more than explanatory devices from which different choices of components and sequences between them can be created as needed. The cycles are good tools, but the adoption of a cyclical sequence and the inclusion of each of these elements are not always necessary to the performance of good audit. A cycle implies certain sequences; it assumes that the end point is always the starting point for the next sequence of actions, and that actions follow each other in a certain order. These assumptions may, but need not, hold true for audit activities.

Possible connections between the patient care cycle, the standards setting cycle, the clinical audit cycle and the change cycle are deployed in Chapter 3 and presented in Figure 7.2. The figure shows how many are the steps to be taken and how complicated are the connections between them when practitioners engage in patient care, standards setting, clinical audit and change.

The standards setting cycle relates to Stage 2 (set standards/goals) of the clinical audit cycle. The connection between the patient care cycle and

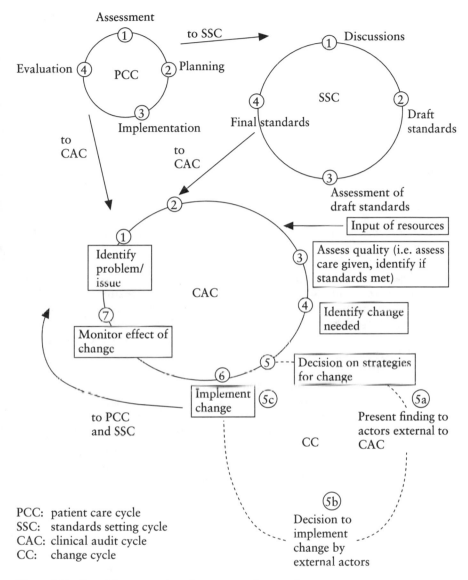

Figure 7.2 Possible connections between various cycles

the clinical audit cycle is likely to occur at Stage 1 of the latter, identifying the problem or issue for audit. The clinical audit cycle may link with the change cycle at Stage 5 (decision on strategies for change) and again at Stage 6 (implement change), depending on whether change is beyond the competence or scope of those engaged in clinical audit and requires a wider group to be engaged in the change.

Any changes affecting clinical care emerging from the clinical audit cycle should feed back to the patient care cycle and to the standards setting cycle. Indeed, each stage of the patient care cycle – assessment, planning, implementation and evaluation – could become a subject for clinical audit in its own right and thus part of a more comprehensive clinical audit cycle.

These connections emerged as findings from our research; we hope they will guide the implementation of clinical audit.

By way of illustration, the example given in the annex to this chapter takes us through each of the seven stages of the clinical audit cycle for one phase of the patient care cycle: assessment. A similar process can be worked through for the other three phases of the patient care cycle.

Outcome analysis

Outcomes, that is, intermediate outcomes, emerge at each phase of the patient care cycle but it is at the evaluation phase when they tend to assume particular importance because they are likely to focus on the patient's health status rather than on processes of care. However, a great deal of patient care evaluation assesses the success of the treatment and so the quality of the process of care is an important outcome too. Intermediate outcomes of processes of care should be linked to the final health status outcome so that professionals can be confident that it was their treatment that led to the final outcome.

A similar argument about intermediate outcomes applies to clinical audit except that audit focuses on the quality of a service rather than the quality of care for individual patients. Data collected from evaluations of patient care naturally raise questions about the quality of the service more generally. Although final outcomes are especially important, there are intermediate outcomes at each stage of the audit process that, in aggregate, contribute to the final outcome. For example, the following problem concerning patient referral times illustrates the outcomes that might occur at each stage of the clinical audit cycle.

The problem: the time between being referred and being seen by a therapist is regarded by clients as too long

Stage 1: identify problem/issue   The outcome of this stage might be awareness by the therapists of the worry experienced by clients waiting to be seen.

Stage 2: set standards   Outcomes are that standards were set and the process of standards setting had a positive effect on staff morale.

Stage 3: assess/measure quality   The assessment of the referral–appointment time lag shows that the standard specified has not been reached but all the staff feel involved and consulted in the process.

Stage 4: identify change needed The therapists agree that, to implement the change needed, evening clinics are necessary and this requires commitment from all members of the multi-professional team.

Stage 5: decision on strategies for change The service manager agrees that unsocial hours payments are justified for evening clinics and confirms that the budget will stand this.

Stage 6: implement change The therapists review their home commitments to accommodate evening clinics. The clinics are introduced on two evenings a week for a trial period of three months.

Stage 7: monitor effect of change The time between referral and being seen by a therapist is less than it was and there are fewer complaints from clients.

There is a danger that the current emphasis on outcome might produce superficial audit, concerned with easily quantifiable final outcomes, rather than more meaningful audit that links process to outcome. Practitioners might be insufficiently connected to either professional or general managers and other organizations, which should have access to audit data, to be able to move from individual patients' outcomes to service outcomes. This means that there are few actual links as yet between the patient care cycle and the clinical audit cycle.

Work on uni-professional outcomes is often concerned with the specialized technical core of each profession. The results of these specialized outcomes could, however, feed into broader multi-professional outcomes. Although they are likely to be less specialized, multi-professional outcomes can be concerned with core clinical activities as practised by a multi-professional care team.

Multiple concerns and multi-professionality

Clinical audit must involve expressing data and knowledge in a form which is communicable outside the auditing and audited group, and there must be systems or mechanisms enabling it to be transmitted and used by outside groups. Audit is intended to yield data that are usable by different groups of stake-holders, for different purposes. The users include the professionals, acting singly or jointly, professional service managers, general provider managers, purchasers, clients and patients. Some will look for specific and measurable outcomes, others for the more complex processual outcomes. Managers and purchasers might seek particular forms of outcome analysis. Among the multiple purposes of audit, managers can use it for the allocation of resources and the monitoring, on behalf of a health unit or authority, of performance and clinical effectiveness. The same data may be used for purposes of self-development and self-knowledge, but to constitute audit, they must have certain institutional characteristics. Later we propose ways in which institutional arrangements can be used to enhance audit.

The nature of audit varies according to which group is driving it. General managers and purchasers are generally more concerned with whole patient services, that is, the generic and systemic layers of quality assurance; their interests are more likely to be met by the results of multi- rather than uni-professional audit.

The primary purpose of clinical audit is the verification of the worth of clinical processes. It has, however, secondary and tertiary purposes to inform judgements on the relationship between clinical work and generic and systemic objectives of the organization (Table 7.1).

The concerns of the professional service manager are linked with the process of care (therefore the technical level of quality assurance) as well as with more generic concerns for the quality of the service as a whole. The professional service manager gives a lead and focus to uni-professional clinical audit. By contrast, multi-professional audit may lack the focus of accountability found in uni-professional audit. To succeed, clear channels of accountability and authority to effect change need to be established above the level of the multi-professional team leader.

Clear and formal connections with general managers and purchasers are needed above the professional service manager level. It is at the junction between the clinical audit cycle and the external change cycle that connections are often lacking, leading to failure to effect change. This leads to demoralization of the providers involved in the audit and lack of impact of the audit data on broader organizational concerns. There is then a need for greater involvement of general management in the audit process, at each step of the clinical audit cycle, so that the process of identifying the change needed and implementing it remains part of the same clinical audit cycle.

Connections are often lacking between purchasers and providers. Providers need to inform and advise purchasers on the core quality issues related to clinical care. Indeed, connections to promote and progress audit are needed at all levels of the organization, and even across organizations, with social services, voluntary organizations and the educational sector.

All of these multiple concerns point to the need for negotiated objectives and operational patterns of clinical audit.

The links between audit and management are two-directional. In the term used frequently in total quality management, audit initiatives are 'top-led and bottom-fed'. The meeting point between systems management and professional work for audit as well as for clinical care will be the professional service manager. The professional service manager serves as the link between the providers and management and purchasers, transmitting data upward and feeding information on results and change back to the providers. Appropriate support, interest and feedback mechanisms from general managers and purchasers to provider level are needed. However, the main thrust and enthusiasm for audit, especially when linked to core

Table 7.1 Connections of clinical audit (for uni- or multi-professional clinical audit)

Essential connections	Organizational level	Mode of quality assurance	Examples of prerequisites
1 Connecting clinical audit cycle with the patient care and standards setting cycles	• intra-service • possibly supra-organizational (e.g. national standards set by professional bodies)	• technical • generic	• clinical knowledge base of professionals • knowledge on audit and quality issues/methods • authority of the professional service manager/team leader to effect change within the service
2 Connecting the four cycles (clinical audit, patient care, standards setting, change cycles)	• essentially intra-service	• technical • generic • systemic	• connections between the professional service manager/team leader and general management • clear lines of accountability for audit
3 Connecting clinical audit with other forms of audit and quality assurance	• intra-service and/or inter-service	• technical • generic • systemic	• unit-wide quality/audit committee ensuring connections between the different groups (quality assurance staff, providers, professional service managers, general managers) • unit-wide data system • clear lines of accountability for audit
4 Connecting clinical audit with purchasers	• intra-service and/or inter-service	• technical • generic • systemic	• unit-wide quality/audit committee, including purchasers • possibly direct connections between purchasers and providers • unit-wide data system • clear lines of accountability for audit
5 Connecting clinical audit with non-health service groups/ organizations	• inter-service	• technical • generic • systemic	• unit-wide quality/audit committee, including representatives from consumers and non-NHS providers and purchasers • clear lines of accountability for audit • cross-organizational data system

clinical issues, need to come from the providers. In order to generate enthusiasm at the working base, it is necessary to give professionals the freedom to use their expertise to select clinical audit topics and carry them out as well as appropriate support.

Sharing audit methods and results across trusts is desirable in order to increase knowledge and build on existing patterns at a national level. Care must be taken that the development of a commercial ethos in the trusts does not impede this process. The professional bodies have a role to play in the dissemination of audit methods and knowledge across trusts, in particular in setting uni-professional standards and devising protocols and outcome measures.

We have noted that clinical audit is primarily concerned with appraisal of clinical work. This feeds into judgements about generic and systemic work. Only perhaps BS5750 is concerned with the appraisal of technical processes. Other forms of quality assurance are primarily concerned with generic and systemic issues. But links between different forms of quality assurance do not emerge as strong. There is a need for unit-wide quality assurance frameworks incorporating the various forms of quality assurance and audit.

Definition of the functions of the whole range of quality assurance – medical audit, clinical audit, BS5750, total quality management, King's Fund Organizational Audit, Patient's Charter and resource management – would be helpful to ensure reduction of overlap and some confusion.

Links with medical audit are growing. In many cases multi-professional audit is led by medical clinicians. Anxieties remain that medical leadership will tend to emphasize particular aspects of clinical care at the expense of process issues related to quality of life. However, there is evidence that medical thinking can be enriched by working within multi-professional settings.

Multi-professional working

Current policy is that clinical audit should be multi-professional. The advantages of multi-professional audits are obvious. Ultimately, care converges upon individual patients or groups within society, and it makes no sense to avoid consideration of the efficacy of one process while performing another. Shared knowledge of both clinical practice and ways of auditing it would avoid waste of resource and effort, and amateurism.

Clinical audit might, however, best begin with professions becoming sufficiently competent in the evaluation of their own work to grasp the content and techniques of clinical audit as it applies to them. They then might look for common elements to be usefully merged into multi-professional, including medical, audit. The best patterns might include hybrid arrangements in which strong uni-professional audit is maintained, but with the merging of those elements that can be beneficially undertaken in common.

It is likely that uni-professional audit will sustain a high technical content. As uni-professional audits move into collaboration with other uni-professional audits, the concerns will become more generic and systemic, and more likely, therefore, to include more comfortably the needs of both management and client groups. This does not mean, of course, that clinical practice undertaken by more than one profession cannot usefully be assessed by a multi-professional audit.

Professionals do not, however, necessarily work as part of a team and some areas of care are best suited to uni-professional audit. And there are differences in the status and ways of working of the professions which mean that multi-professional audit needs, in some cases, to be approached carefully. Another important factor making for differences is that some specialties or client groups are more suited to multi-professional audit than others. Clinical audit is intended to enhance clinical effectiveness, a task which will be best promoted by uni- or multi-professional audit depending on the situation or, indeed, a combination of both.

It is these considerations, the imperatives imposed by ways of working together, which underlie our proposals for mandating and mechanisms below.

Mandating

Mandating takes place at three levels: the creation of machinery at the unit/trust level; the incorporation of the principal working groups into that machinery, in which the role of the professional service managers is crucial; and the internalization of audit by individual practitioners.

Quality assurance in general is often thought to lack a clear mandate from the top. The trust and chief executive must therefore sponsor it as an essential part of the development and monitoring capacity of the unit. This includes the need to encourage the work of professional managers in pursuing issues of clinical effectiveness and in ensuring that a concern for process is also encouraged in quality assurance, including audit.

Machinery

The machinery of audit and its resource implications must be considered at the unit, professional service and individual levels.

The unit level

Audit evokes two sets of sponsors. The professions must take primary ownership of audit. But its good development also concerns unit management in their pursuit of managerial and clinical effectiveness. There might be a conflict between these concerns; negotiation between professional-clinical and systems-managerial positions will be necessary.

Mandating and sponsorship can then be articulated by the creation of a unit committee linking the two interests, taking system-wide responsibility for audit and incorporating professional representation. This committee may be part of a quality assurance committee whose concerns include clinical audit. The committee should contain full representation from the levels of the chief executive, directors of services, the main professions and the purchasers. Its reports should be available to the trust board as well as professional managers and practitioners. It is of crucial importance that a full spectrum of professionals involved in clinical audit are represented on the committee. In some cases, there may be a need to create sub-committees at directorate or clinical team level. Proper feedback mechanisms need to be established between the various committees, and the unit committee and the providers. The professional service manager or an audit or quality facilitator may be the best person to ensure these connections.

The unit committee should act both executively and deliberatively. It should engage in systematic agenda building in which the emphasis is on development rather than control.

The committee's agendas might contain items of the following kind:

- receiving and giving feedback on reports on the ways in which professional groups are developing audit
- encouraging and receiving reports on specific audit projects, which might also entail progress chasing in view of the requirements of purchasers for evidence of audit
- evaluating audit methodologies: the role of professionals on the committee will be central in ensuring that audit questions inform research and vice versa
- deciding how the total organization can better facilitate audit, and ensuring linkage between clinical, generic and systemic modes of audit: in particular, ensuring linkage between relevant data sources in the unit
- ensuring linkage with other quality initiatives (medical audit, if still separate, total quality management, Patient's Charter, BS5750)
- supporting the professional groups in their audit initiatives
- determining resources for audit
- allocating resources for audit
- determining unit-wide audit training needs and ways of meeting them
- providing technical and other audit support to the professional groups
- ensuring that recommended actions have been taken.

The professional service level
The main action required in undertaking clinical audit will rest with the professionals within their groupings. It is there that the expertise lies.

In some cases, clinical audit might develop across units as the result of professional initiatives, although this is likely to become more difficult with the organization of the health service into trusts. In other cases, clinical audit might develop in direct collaboration between purchasers and professionals, thus linking the systemic and technical aspects of quality assurance. These developments are to be encouraged by the unit audit committee if they promote clinical effectiveness. However, all main audit initiatives need to be discussed and reported to the committee in order to ensure coordination and to gain maximum support and impact.

The professional service manager is at the interface between the interests and concerns of professionals and those of general management. S/he plays a crucial role in accomplishing audit and effecting change. Hence, it is necessary to ensure that, at unit level, there is support and stability of employment for professional service managers, and that some time is built into the contracts of professional service managers for them to initiate and maintain audit.

The main points for action by the professional service manager and his/her staff are:

- make the main decisions concerning the content of audit: the professional service manager may emphasize professional concerns with technicity and genericism, as well as managerial concerns
- make timetables for audit development
- allocate specific time for developing audit procedures: specific time allocation for audit may need to be built into the work contracts of professionals, taking into account their degrees of involvement in clinical audit
- make judgements on the connections to be made with the other professions in order to identify those parts of audit that are to be specialist and uni-professional and those that can/should be multi-professional
- make judgements and take decisions on the connections to be made with general managers and purchasers in order to effect the change identified as necessary by the audit
- evaluate the results of audit in terms of patient care performance and planning
- ensure that audit results are appropriately fed back to all staff concerned, to general managers and to purchasers
- ensure that audit is integrated in the training of professionals
- seek installation of appropriate information technology facilities and ensure compatibility with the unit system of data collection: this will mean ensuring adequate facilities for capturing and analysing data as well as appropriate support to use them.

The individual level
If professionals are to move beyond compliance to commitment to audit, it needs to become internalized by individuals and become part of normal professional practice. In order to achieve this, audit needs to be mandated by the professions, NHS management and training.

Audit is a part of professional responsibility, but it is also a way to self-development in the key professional tasks. Its use invokes particular modes of behaviour, such as gaining consensus on the best use of time at meetings by inviting members to review the conduct and progress of the meetings periodically.

Issues of confidentiality related to the care of patients and between professionals must be respected. This will help openness between the main stake-holders (providers, patients, purchasers, general managers) and willingness on the part of the professionals to tackle sensitive quality issues.

Resources

Several kinds of resources are needed for successful audit:

- a considered time allowance for professionals and others engaged in audit
- relatively small sums of money for stationery, printing and the like. This money might come initially from the unit, but it will be operationally and symbolically appropriate for addition to be made to the budgets of operating groups so that audit becomes fully integrated into their professional working
- information technology resources, if competent and aggregatable data are to be gathered and manipulated. Many professionals will need technical training in their use. This initiative needs to be linked, at unit level, to other resource management initiatives
- clerical support
- clinical audit staff, providing advice and help with audit activities, to support professional groups in gaining expertise on the purposes, methods and exploitation of audit procedures
- a person skilled in data analysis and computer systems providing technical support to the different professional groups in varying degrees according to need, and ensuring that technical issues are successfully handled
- stable and long-term employment for audit staff so that continuity of support for professionals is ensured.

These propositions and suggestions should thus be regarded as possibilities to be taken up by professionals as contributions to their own modelling.

An evaluative matrix

Evaluation is the underlying activity of audit and underpins many of its stages. It is also important, however, to evaluate the impact of audit on policy, organization and practice.

In Table 7.2 we offer a matrix of the modes of audit and of the factors which might enhance, or otherwise, audit activities. This would have the two uses of evaluating the strategy for clinical audit in the organization and evaluating the effects of change on the organization of the clinical audit strategy.

The matrix might be read as follows. The many factors influencing how audit is carried out appear in the vertical axis. It is worthwhile for those

Table 7.2 An evaluative matrix for clinical audit

Some factors influencing mode of audit	Modes of audit			
	Uni-professional	*Multi-professional*	*Core activities*	*Non-core activities*
• setting – acute/community				
• client group				
• directorate structure	2/1	5		
• unit-wide committee				
• linkage between clinical audit and other forms of audit/quality assurance				
• direct linkage between purchasers and providers	3	3	2	4
• linkage between the provider level and general management				
• linkage between the provider unit and other agencies				
• linkage with user groups				
• clear lines of accountability for audit at all levels of the organization				
• authority to act on audit results				
• use of audit results in allocation of resources				
• time built in				
• audit staff				
• availability of data systems with unit-wide compatibility				
• data systems compatibility across organizations (inter-trusts, inter-NHS/social service)				
• audit as a means of professional development and continuing education for staff				
• audit as a means of staff appraisal and monitoring				

involved in audit to augment this list to take account of their own circumstances. The list can then be used to judge how far the factors affect the
modes of audit shown in the horizontal axis. This would enable general
and professional managers to assess the extent to which their arrangements enhance audit activities. It would strengthen the rigour of the exercise if these relationships were graded (1 = no relationship, 5 = very strong
relationship), although such gradings should be used only for purposes of
illuminating discussion. For example, a unit audit committee might consider whether its move towards a directorate structure enhances strongly
(5) multi-professional and weakens (2 or 1) uni-professional audit. A professional manager might consider whether stronger links between purchasers and providers could support equally either uni- or multi-professional
audit (3) whilst encouraging non-core modes of audit (4) at the expense
of core activities (2).

Conclusion

Audit can take on several styles and summon many different responses. It
should be seen primarily as a device for self-monitoring and enhancing the
development of professional self-confidence and status. At the same time
it can provide a fair basis for accountability and managerial monitoring.
We hope this book shows the way to professionals who wish to take
ownership of a movement which will certainly add to their work but also
enhance the contribution that they can make to the health services.

Annex: an example of linkage between the clinical audit cycle and the assessment stage of the patient care cycle

We give here an example of linkage between the clinical audit cycle and
the assessment stage of the patient care cycle.

First, though, we describe the patient care cycle for the patient who is
an elderly woman with memory problems and periodic disorientation and
anxiety who is referred to the clinical psychology service by the GP.

The patient care cycle

Phase 1: assessment   The clinical psychologist visits the patient at home
and assesses the existence and extent of her memory and orientation problems using observation and a standard scale the effect of these problems
on her ability to continue to cope at home alone.

Phase 2: planning   The goals agreed by the psychologist and the patient
are that her anxiety will decrease and her independence will increase within
one month. The plan of care is negotiated with the patient and her daughter and includes:

- increasing cues in the patient's environment to jog her memory and maximize her independence
- arranging social services support (home help and meals on wheels three times a week)
- reducing risks to her safety and increasing her daughter's peace of mind (an emergency button linked to a central monitoring service, a telephone call from her daughter every morning).

The psychologist writes to the GP outlining this care plan and requesting referral to a community psychiatric nurse to plan details of the proposed programme, implement it and monitor the patient's progress.

Phase 3: implementation   The plan of care is put in motion by the nurse.

Phase 4: evaluation   The psychologist and nurse together assess whether the plan of care was executed and the goals achieved. They adjust the goals and care plan accordingly and set a date for further evaluation.

We can now describe what the seven stages of the clinical audit cycle might look like at the assessment phase of the patient care cycle (see Figure 7.3).

Example of a clinical audit cycle at the assessment phase of the patient care cycle

Stage 1: identify problem/issue   The clinical psychology service has received complaints from patients' relatives that psychologists' interpersonal communication style with patients is inadequate during the assessment process so that patients underperform; the result is an inaccurate outcome of the psychologists' assessments.

Stage 2: set standards   All the clinical psychologists in the service agree the standard: that their interpersonal communication style will not adversely affect a client's performance.

Stage 3: assess/measure quality   Video recordings are made of a random selection of psychologists' assessment meetings with clients. Independent peers judge the adequacy of interpersonal communication and they confirm that the standard is not being met.

Stage 4: identify change needed   General changes identified are that the duration of each client assessment session will be increased from 30 to 40 minutes. Two of the clinical psychologists would benefit from attending a course that focuses on interpersonal communication skills.

Stage 5: decisions on strategy for change   It is agreed that:

1 client appointments will be rescheduled
2 the contract with purchasers will be renegotiated to allow for greater assessment time per client

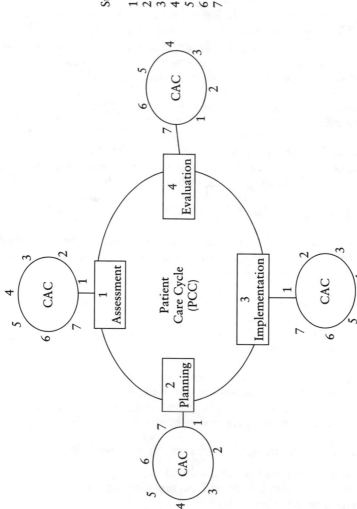

Stages of the clinical audit cycle (CAC)

1 identify problem/issue
2 set standards
3 assess/measure quality
4 identify change needed
5 decision on strategies for change
6 implement change
7 monitor effect of change

Figure 7.3 Clinical audit cycles at each phase of the patient care cycle

3 money will be earmarked for interpersonal communication skills courses for clinical psychologists who need help.

Stage 6: implement change   This stage asks whether the decisions taken in Stage 5 were implemented. In this case decisions 1 and 2 were discussed with the clinical psychologists' professional manager (so entering the change cycle depicted in Figure 7.2). Decision 3 is implemented by the psychologists from their education budget.

Stage 7: monitor effect of change   This final stage of the clinical audit cycle asks whether the plan worked. This is done by continuing to monitor the number of complaints received about the adequacy of psychologists' interpersonal communication style when assessing clients. If the number of complaints is zero and the standard set is reached then no further action is required. If problems remain, or new ones emerge, then the clinical audit cycle is set in motion once again.

These mini cycles at each stage of the patient care cycle can then become incorporated in a larger clinical audit cycle that addresses the clinical psychology service more widely.

Appendix 1
Members of the clinical audit advisory group

Paddy Bateson, District Speech Therapist/Clinical Audit Coordinator, Walton Hospital, Chesterfield.

Dr Mike Berger, District Psychologist, St George's Healthcare, London.

John Brennan, Head of Quality Support Centre, The Open University Quality Support Services, London.

Dr John Cape, Psychology Services Manager, Camden and Islington Community Health Services NHS Trust, London.

Christine Chalmers, Manager of Speech and Language Therapy Services, St Martin's Hospital, Bath.

Anna Farrer, Speech and Language Therapy Services Manager, Dacorum and St Albans Community NHS Trust, St Albans.

Sally Gore, Director of Primary Health Care, Southampton Community Health Services.

Professor Robert Harris, Department of Social Work, University of Hull.

Ann Hunter, formerly Director of Therapy, Guy's Hospital, London, now Project Manager, Ninewells Hospital and Medical School, Dundee.

Jane Langley, Professional Affairs Consultant, The Chartered Society of Physiotherapy, from August 1992 to November 1992.

Rita Patel, formerly Team Manager, Rehabilitation and Continuing Care, the Keyham Centre, Towers Hospital, Leicester, now Service Unit Manager for Clinical Support Services, Edith Cavell Hospital, Peterborough, from November 1992.

Trish Phillips, Chairman of Council, The Chartered Society of Physiotherapy, from August 1992 to March 1993.

Sheelagh Richards, Occupational Therapy Officer representing all the participating professions, Department of Health.

Karen Romain, Senior Professional Affairs Officer, The Chartered Society of Physiotherapy, from November 1992.

Beryl Steeden, Director of Professional Affairs, College of Occupational Therapists, from August 1992 to November 1992.

Appendix 2
The methods used in the study

Sarah Robinson and Maurice Kogan

A full account of the methods used in our study can be found in our final report to the Department of Health (Redfern *et al.* 1995). Here we give an abridged version.

Aims of the project

The aims of the project, as agreed at the outset with our Department of Health customers, were twofold: first, to document and analyse examples of audit practice in the four professions, and second, to produce guidelines on models of good practice, upon which the four professions might base their audit activities in the future; in particular to identify whether a common core of components existed that might form the basis of a framework for multi-professional audit.

Our remit thus required us to engage in two different kinds of activity: discovery of existing states of quality audit – a task for systematic enquiry – and the development of models of clinical audit that might guide policy makers and practitioners in the future. These two activities of discovery and development were undertaken by means of a five-phase project.

Phase 1: preliminary work

Preliminary work included the overall design of the five-phase operational programme of research and development, together with detailed plans for the events to be undertaken within each phase. Project staff were appointed, and the Nursing and Therapy Audit Networks were joined to facilitate identification of possible sites for fieldwork. An advisory group was set up. The literature was reviewed as part of the process of formulating research questions and delineating contexts in which the work was to be based.

Phase 2: design of instruments and selection of sites

Phase 2 of the project comprised three activities: interviews with key informants, selection of the case study sites, and developing interview schedules and the range of interviewees.

Interviews with key informants

Interviews were held in the early weeks of Phase 2 with ten key informants drawn from the four professions. The interviews focused on the following themes concerning the development and practice of audit:

- the informants' own definitions of audit and of clinical audit, and the way(s) in which these terms were used in their profession
- work on standards setting at national and local level and the extent to which these were compatible with purchaser guidelines
- the history of the development of audit in the professions, the initiatives and impetus for development and the way in which audit principles and practice had been shaped over time
- views about the Normand Report and developments in audit activities since its publication
- the informants' own involvement in audit activities
- the stage of development in the profession in relation to defining and measuring outcomes of practice and outcomes of audit
- the impact on audit activities of the NHS reforms and of various types of service organization, e.g. clinical directorates
- views on desirability and feasibility of multi-professional audit in the professions
- actual and desired links between audit in the professions and medical and nursing audit
- the outcomes they would like to see emerging from this project.

The key informant interviews provided a wealth of material about audit.

Selection of case study sites

It was not feasible for sites to be representative of the state of audit development in England. It was, however, essential that a diversity of audit activity and context be represented in a purposively chosen sample of sites. Consequently a detailed process of identification, evaluation and consultation took place in order that this diversity be achieved.

The criteria for site selection were: an active history of audit, geographical spread, representation of professions, setting (to include audit in hospital and in community settings), organization client group, and keenness to participate.

Consultation with the advisory group

A list of 12 sites was sent to the professional members of the advisory group for comments on their suitability or otherwise. Members of the group had circulated news of the research widely among their own professions and this had produced information about projects that had not been identified by the National Nursing and Therapy Audit Network and the regional audit coordinators. A revised list of sites was drawn up that included some from the first list, plus some recommended by members of the advisory group.

In making a final selection from the revised list, the question of including sites in which members of the advisory group were involved had to be resolved. It was decided not to include in the main fieldwork those sites in which advisory group members were based, but rather to select three for inclusion in additional fieldwork, in which our findings and models could be tested.

The identity of the nine sites remained confidential to the research team and the advisory group.

Developing interview schedules and range of interviewees

Interviews constituted the main component of fieldwork; they were undertaken in order to learn about the state of audit as experienced by those in the field, and to obtain their perceptions on its progress and effectiveness. The following range of personnel was identified for inclusion:

- therapists holding primarily clinical posts
- therapists holding primarily managerial posts
- nurses working with therapists
- doctors working with therapists
- business/general managers at unit level
- chief executive of the trust
- quality adviser(s) at different levels: unit/district/region/service
- district general manager/purchasing manager
- director of public health
- regional audit adviser/coordinator.

Members of the four professions constituted the largest group of interviewees at each site. Most meetings were individual.

Content of interview schedules
The main themes were:

- structure of health service organization of the site, and interviewees' place within it
- definitions of audit and clinical audit
- history of audit at different levels of health service organization: region/district/provider units/therapy profession
- identification of principles that guide audit and standards setting
- professional and management agenda for audit: extent to which people at different levels of organization were involved in formulating the agenda
- process and outcomes measures used in assessment of care provided
- methods used in carrying out audit (e.g. discussion of case notes, analysis of critical incidents, monitoring key indicators, criterion-based audit)
- management of audit process and specification of outcomes
- existence and perceived adequacy of uni- and multi-professional audit tools, and whether they were based on existing scales or measures or devised for a specific project
- responsibility for ensuring audit takes place
- impact of purchasers' requirements on audit
- resources required and resources available for audit

- perceived effect of audit on care delivery and on professional education and development, particularly translation of audit findings into professional and managerial decisions
- links of audit in the professions with medical audit and nursing audit, and links between audit and other forms of quality assurance (for example, total quality management, King's Fund audit, BS5750, peer review)
- factors that facilitate or constrain the development and progress of audit
- views on feasibility of a multi-professional framework for audit.

An interview schedule for each of the types of personnel was drafted, drawing on the themes listed above as appropriate.

Drafting and piloting
The draft schedules were circulated to the advisory group. Following minor revisions made in the light of the group's comments, the schedules were piloted. The interview schedules for therapists were the longest and most complex of the ten; they were also the cornerstone of the fieldwork. All schedules were piloted with representatives of the groups listed above.

Phase 3: fieldwork

Phase 3 of the project entailed fieldwork in the six main sites. During the process of site selection the key person had been identified with whom access should be negotiated. A letter of request was followed up by a telephone call. The letter outlined the purpose of the project, the reasons why the particular site had been selected for inclusion and a request for participation. Response from all six sites indicated a willingness to participate. Personnel at two sites, however, requested a meeting with team members for further discussion before committing themselves.

Access meetings were then arranged at each site. The research team received a warm welcome at the six meetings, and help in planning fieldwork, although expectations varied as to what the team would in turn bring to the site.

A programme of interviews was arranged once agreement had been reached on the audit projects to be studied and the people to be interviewed. Assurances of confidentiality were given, and a request made to bring written documentation about audit activities to the interview. Site personnel were immensely helpful in both organizing a fieldwork schedule that used our time as efficiently as possible, and in driving us to the various locations involved.

Interviews

The majority of the interviews lasted about an hour. Those with therapists in management positions usually took longer, since the interview focused on both the professional and managerial aspects of their role in relation to audit. Some interviewees were initially quite guarded in their responses; this was especially likely at sites in the throes of organizational change and concomitant uncertainty about roles in the new structure. Initial reservation was also encountered with some of the therapists working in situations in which audit had been managerially rather than professionally generated. In nearly all cases, however, initial hesitancies were overcome and conversation flowed freely. At the end of the interview, many expressed surprise that they had talked for so long; as one said, 'I would never have thought I had so much to say about audit.'

Another frequent comment at the end of the interview was an admission of nervousness prior to the event; the team had been perceived as 'assessors', rather than as researchers coming to learn about the progress of audit as experienced by those most closely involved.

Data handling

A comprehensive account of the interview was produced by the interviewer as soon as possible after the event. The account was structured under the headings of the interview schedule and included significant verbatims. Each section of text was numbered to correspond with the schedule. Producing these accounts was a lengthy undertaking, of often up to three hours per interview. The interviews were entered into a computer database using a program called File Maker. This provided the facility of printing out all those sections of text relating to a particular topic.

We worked in nine sites in all; the six main study sites and the additional three for preliminary model testing. Developing future models took precedence over describing the state of clinical audit in England. The sample was weighted inasmuch as all had achieved some progress with audit. Although the method employed did not attempt to establish a comprehensive empirical base, 122 people were interviewed in the six sites and information obtained about over 100 audit activities of varying kinds. On the basis of fieldwork, together with reading of the literature, we moved to the second element of the research, namely the development and testing of models of good practice.

Phase 4: analysis and model development

Phase 4 of the research comprised both data analysis and model development. The fieldwork in the six sites revealed diversity and complexity of both audit activities and views concerning the development of audit generally. As we immersed ourselves in this material we also moved to our developmental objective. Testing emerging models and concepts, followed by further development and clarification, were integral parts of the project design.

The aim of our analysis was to move from the detail of events and views in six specific case study sites to a range of models and guidelines that could be adapted for use in a variety of health care settings. None the less it was apparent from the start of fieldwork that the development of audit activities had first to be analysed in the context of the site in which they were based, since their particular form was to some extent determined by that context. Consequently a thorough understanding of each case study was necessary before moving to models and other commonalities. After completion of fieldwork at each site, therefore, a detailed site report was produced. This process of site analysis entailed careful verification of interviewces' responses against written documents.

After completion of fieldwork in two sites, we started the process of disaggregating and reaggregating the components of audit; this work had two main strands: first, a series of cycles concerned with:

- providing individual patient/client care
- standards setting
- auditing care and service organization
- implementing changes indicated by the audit.

This work was also concerned with the ways in which these cycles link with each other. The second strand addressed the key elements of audit, which were identified as:

- categories of audit
- the connection of clinical audit with management
- relationship of audit with other quality assurance activities
- the impact of audit on delivery of care, on service organization and on professional development of individuals, and the factors that facilitate or constrain its progress.

Both the development of the cycles, and the delineation of the key elements of audit drew on two units of analysis: the specific audit activities in progress (or completed), and individual members of site staff.

Moving from these units of analysis to the cycles and to the key elements of audit necessitated an intermediate stage of mapping the data on to charts. Each activity was mapped in relation to its initiation, focus, personnel involved, organizational links, level of maturity and impact. Responses made by individuals were mapped by the topics covered by the schedules. For each topic this process enabled us to ascertain the themes that emerged, and the range of experiences and views expressed in relation to each theme.

The aim of the project was not to produce precise quantification in the sense of 'twenty people said this, whereas twenty-five said that . . .'. Rather it was to demonstrate the issues that are important to the development of clinical audit in both uni- and multi-professional contexts, whether they came within the experience of the majority of respondents or not. In the chapters in which findings are presented we have not given many numbers, but have indicated whether the experiences or views under consideration held good for a majority (all, most, many), a substantial minority (some, several) or for just a few individuals.

Initial testing of models

Our developing models, which at this stage consisted of the cycles and the connections between them, were tested internally and externally. For *internal testing*, the models were continually tested by the team against the data from the six case study sites. For *external testing*, limited though intensive fieldwork was undertaken in the three further sites. At each of these, two members of the research team spent up to a day working with site personnel. The 29 who attended represented each of the four professions, together with members of other professions, holders of quality assurance posts and managers. In the first part of the meeting, information was presented about audit activities in progress at the site; this provided a context for the second part of the meeting, in which our findings and models were tested against the situation at the site and the views and experiences of those attending. Overall our models seemed in accord with their perceptions and experiences of audit, although a number of modifications were suggested.

Reformulation of models and further analysis of data

The models were reformulated in the light of the internal and external testing that we had undertaken. This reformulation entailed both modelling of connections between cycles and normative modelling in which we moved towards guidelines for the professions.

Final testing of models

This final stage of testing entailed discussion with members of the advisory group at its final meeting. Following the outcome of this event, the models' framework and guidelines, presented in Chapter 7, were made final.

Phase 5: dissemination

The last phase of the project is entailing a programme of dissemination. From the outset of the work, Department of Health customers and members of the advisory group attached considerable importance to making findings widely available to members of the professions and to health service managers.

The project in retrospect

The project constitutes an unusual approach to research and development. Policy analysis of the kind attempted here cannot depend wholly on empirical discovery. It does require discovery of existing states, but then a creative leap into conjectural analysis of likely feasible patterns for further action. The patterns should then be tested against the experiences of practitioners, managers and policy makers. The process in this project has been one of immersion in states of clinical audit in 1993 and 1994, with documentation and analysis of the complexity existing at that time. This has been followed by attempts at creative modelling and provision of guidelines upon which the professions can base their audit activities in future.

Appendix 3
The development of an audit culture in the four professions

Anémone Kober and Sally Redfern

The role of the professional bodies

All health care professions are influenced by their national bodies, whose role in developing clinical audit is central. For one thing, the professional bodies have an important role in proposing and validating standards of training and in promoting quality issues. We know that the College of Occupational Therapists (COT), the Chartered Society of Physiotherapy (CSP) and the College of Speech and Language Therapists (CSLT) are active in promoting multi-professional collaboration whilst reorganizing the unique contribution of each profession. Their multi-professional endeavours centre on assessment, planning and management of clinical care and also on clinical audit and outcome measurement (CSLT, COT, CSP undated).

The British Psychological Society (BPS)

The professional status of psychology is not at present bound by statute. The BPS recently introduced a charter in an attempt to control the quality of psychologist practice. Application for chartered status is voluntary at present (Management Advisory Service 1989).

The College of Occupational Therapists

In 1974, two bodies combined to form the British Association of Occupational Therapists (BAOT), an independently listed trade union, with the College responsible for professional and educational matters. The College specifies standards of entry to training, curricula, qualifying examinations and codes of ethics for practitioners. The organization's Code of Professional Conduct (revised in 1990) serves to 'promote voluntary standards of professional behaviour' (British Association of Occupational Therapists 1990). The College is used as a focal point and a source of reference and guidance by occupational therapists.

The Chartered Society of Physiotherapy

The Society was originally founded in 1894 by nurses and midwives as the Society of Trained Masseuses. The Royal Charter was granted in 1970 when the name changed to The Society of Massage and Medical Gymnastics. In 1942 it became The Chartered Society of Physiotherapy and in 1985 it merged with the Society of Remedial Gymnastics. The CSP became an independent trade union in 1976. The Society is active in promoting quality standards.

The College of Speech and Language Therapists

The College of Speech and Language Therapists promotes activities and projects in relation to quality and audit. Following a recent structural reorganization in consultation with members, a strategic plan was developed. The need for standards and regulation within the profession was identified and a voluntary registration scheme was established. On registration, speech and language therapists are expected to comply with the code of conduct and standards of care contained in *Communicating Quality* (CSLT 1991). The role of the College is developing into that of a professional consultancy service. The College can carry out service reviews and external audits by invitation; it offers advice on audit, and is now developing a system of accreditation for speech and language therapy services.

Standards setting and guidelines: national initiatives

Quality assurance started to be considered seriously by the therapy professions at the beginning of the 1980s. In 1983, the European member states of the World Health Organization set up a working group to develop a strategy for introducing quality assurance in the health sector. As a result of the recommendations of this working group, various initiatives were taken, including the King's Fund quality initiative in 1984 (Ellis and Whittington 1993). Since the mid-1980s, the professional bodies have been involved in setting national standards for achieving high quality patient care. Work with the King's Fund in the late 1980s helped some of them to define the basis for standards setting which involved widespread consultation with therapists so that consensus could be reached.

How to define and distinguish between standards, guidelines and criteria is the subject of some debate. Clinical psychology, unlike the other professions, uses guidelines rather than standards and defines them differently (Cape 1991). Guidelines represent general statements of expected quality but are not measurable without further specification, whereas standards are particular components of quality that have been defined.

Clinical psychology

The recent move of psychologists to chartered status generated guidelines for professional practice (BPS 1990), which are sufficiently general to accommodate changes in practice. There are 18 guidelines, including fitness to practise, personal conduct, maintaining confidentiality, administrative responsibility, supervisory responsibility, responsibility for the transmission of skills, advising other professions in the conduct of research and obligations to society, both to one's own and to other professions. A great deal of emphasis is placed on how the clinical psychology profession relates to its environment through direct or indirect contact (research publications).

The BPS working party on quality assurance produced draft guidelines, *Quality Issues in Clinical Psychology* (BPS 1989), which set out general principles of quality assurance and a framework for clinical psychology. These are being revised. The framework takes the form of a matrix using the familiar dimensions of structure, process and outcome, and also 'congruence' (harmony between practitioners and clients and across specialties and organizational levels) and 'quality assurance' (support, monitoring and evaluation activities). These dimensions are included in quality considerations at each interface level: client/practitioner, practitioner/service specialty, service specialty/district and the interface with 'higher level forces' that have an impact on the services (e.g. health authority policies, regional or national guidelines). The guidelines include questions to be addressed by practitioners and psychology managers with reference to their quality assurance activities at each interface level.

Occupational therapy

In recent years, the development of clinical audit in occupational therapy has been influenced by various factors, principal among which has been the quality assurance movement encouraged by the Department of Health and enhanced through the national funding mechanism for audit.

In 1986, the College of Occupational Therapists set up a quality assurance working party which identified the approach for its activities as following Donabedian's (1980) structure, process and outcome framework. The working party developed a set of guidelines to assist therapists in their standards setting endeavours.

In 1989, the College published the first of its series on standards of practice (COT 1989) which gives standards for practice with different types of user (with physical disabilities, with learning disabilities, mentally ill, and those living in their own homes) and refers to six stages in the process of care (referral, assessment, treatment planning, treatment implementation, discharge, reassessment). The standards documents are intended as practice guidelines with the aim of helping to standardize treatment protocols (Ellis and Whittington 1993).

Along with the standards is guidance on quality assurance, on outcomes and on staff performance review and continuing education. It is recommended that quality and outcomes of the service provided are reviewed using methods such as peer review, multidisciplinary discussions and quality circles.

Physiotherapy

The Chartered Society of Physiotherapy responded to the demand for a national framework for good practice for all areas of physiotherapy. A quality assurance working party was set up in 1989, following a workshop and survey of local initiatives on quality issues. The working party was successful in raising awareness among Chartered Society members and in stimulating and facilitating clinical interest groups to produce guidelines or standards for their specific areas of physiotherapy.

Standards for the common core subjects were produced, after consultation, by the working party, together with standards for those areas which were not covered by a clinical interest group. This work resulted in the production of the Chartered

Society of Physiotherapy's *Standards of Physiotherapy Practice* pack in 1990 consisting of a ring-binder containing the core standards and seven clinical interest group booklets. More have been published since and are reviewed every two years. The core standards were last revised in 1993.

The standards are intended as a guide for developing local standards and a tool for clinical audit. Each standard is accompanied by measurable criteria. The second edition of *Standards of Physiotherapy Practice* contains six sections on communication and team work, documentation, assessment, informed consent, environment health and safety, and quality assurance.

Quality assurance in physiotherapy provides 'a systematic method of evaluating the quality of physiotherapy services and [facilitating] continuous improvement' (CSP 1993). The five standards within the quality assurance section cover the framework for activity, user satisfaction, staff participation, key indicators of quality and confidentiality.

An information pack recently produced for members contains the standards; a glossary of terms; references for quality assurance, audit, standards setting and outcome measures; how to set standards, measure consumer satisfaction and implement audit; and a network of physiotherapists who are using outcome measures (CSP 1994).

Speech and language therapy

In 1991, after widespread consultation, the College of Speech and Language Therapists published *Communicating Quality*, its professional standards. These underpin development of local standards for speech and language therapy services and are intended to inform purchasers as well as providers.

According to the College most services have set their own standards and audit takes place in many of these services. The methods most commonly used include case note audit and peer review. The College requires that all services have written plans and case notes, monitor their activities and re-evaluate cases.

Moving beyond standards

The four professions have moved a great deal beyond standards setting towards auditing their activities. Audit training helped to create an audit culture among managers and therapists early on but it was not long before this training initiative was seen to have outgrown its purpose for established therapists. New therapists may not receive much training although they are expected to continue the audit culture already developed. This problem, mentioned to us in relation to speech and language therapy, is also true of the other professions.

A handbook on audit for physiotherapy, occupational therapy and speech and language therapy gives advice on carrying out audit that encompasses the structure, process and outcome of a service (Merrall *et al.* 1991; Farrer *et al.* 1994). There is considerable interest in outcome measurement and the second edition includes a review of work on outcomes and outcome measurement in the therapy professions, and an introduction to multi-professional audit (Farrer *et al.* 1994).

Appendix 4 describes audit activities within clinical psychology, occupational therapy, physiotherapy and speech and language therapy that have been published recently. Here we summarize the areas for audit that have interested the professions before looking at efforts made to establish multi- as well as uni-professional clinical audit activity.

The education and training of clinical psychologists prepare them well for the design and implementation of research methodologies that can be used for audit purposes. But Normand *et al.* (1991a) note that audit in clinical psychology is not highly developed and that audit projects tend to be localized with little systematic fertilization across the profession.

The usefulness of clinical audit of psychotherapy services has been questioned because of the difficulty of disentangling numerous factors that influence outcome (Fonagy and Higgnitt 1989). These authors recommend a comprehensive evaluation of psychotherapy services and a centrally maintained database. Their recommendation materialized in the MRC/NHS Collaborative Psychotherapy Project set up to guide clinical practice, inform theory and report to managers on the efficacy of psychotherapy (Halstead *et al.* 1990).

As Appendix 4 shows, areas of interest to clinical psychologists have been measurement of user satisfaction, multi-professional clinical audit in psychiatric rehabilitation and psychogeriatrics, and uni-professional clinical audit in treatments specific to clinical psychology, such as lithium treatment.

Occupational therapists have been active in multi-professional audit in stroke rehabilitation and in outcome measurement: for example, measures of functional ability and activities of daily living and handicap.

Physiotherapists have used peer review to monitor patient assessment, goal setting and outcome achieved. There has been an interest in outcome measurement, such as quality of life measures, mobility scales and patient satisfaction. Recent work has focused on linking structure and process to outcome to demonstrate the effectiveness of physiotherapy.

As a small profession, development of an audit culture in speech and language therapy may be relatively easy because rapid networking amongst all speech and language therapists in the NHS is a realistic proposition. Their activities have included assessment of care provision across districts and development of outcome measures for specific therapy treatments (e.g. communication ability of aphasic patients) and for multi-professional activities in impairment, disability, handicap and distress. As with the other professions, speech and language therapists have put user feedback high on their agenda in the form of satisfaction surveys.

Appendix 4
A brief review of published audit activities in the four professions

Anémone Kober and Sally Redfern

Audit activities in clinical psychology

User satisfaction

Clinical psychologists have investigated ways in which consumers can be involved in making decisions about services at many different levels (Bell 1991). Studies of patient/user/consumer satisfaction reflect methodological problems associated with these surveys, such as high levels of reported satisfaction, socially desirable or acquiescent responses, and low response rates (Dagnan and Fish 1991; Jenkins and Jakes 1991; McAuliffe and MacLachlan 1992; Larner *et al.* 1993). It has been noted that reported satisfaction may not be as accurate a measure of therapy outcome as asking patients to evaluate their therapy relative to their original problem (Brunning 1992).

Multi-professional clinical audit

Multi-professional audit is advocated for psychiatric rehabilitation (Perkins *et al.* 1992) and mental health settings generally. The QUARTZ system is a team approach that focuses on provision of high quality care in ways informed by knowledge of good practice, the values of the organization and views of users, staff and management (Clifford *et al.* 1992). QUARTZ overcomes the limitations of standard assessment instruments that are not sensitive to small changes in outcome.

Another example of multi-professional audit involving clinical psychology is the Clinical Planning Audit System (CPAS). This was developed to increase the quality of mental health care in a psychogeriatric unit by integrating new initiatives (the care programme approach, case management, the named nurse/key worker concept and discharge planning) into routine care (Riordan and Mockler 1994). Data collection used multi-professional care plans, clinical measures of symptom change and consumer questionnaires. Identification of service deficiencies led to methods for corrective action, such as audit review, case studies, informal feedback and presentation to purchasers to improve joint planning and future planning, thus completing the audit cycle.

Uni-professional clinical audit

Clinical psychologists are also active in uni-professional audit. For example, an audit of lithium screening and monitoring led to development of a revised lithium treatment protocol with accompanying standards, an improved information strategy for clients and clinicians and a video for clients in acute wards and day units (Mason *et al.* 1994). The group plans to extend the new strategy to the primary care sector, thus improving its liaison with secondary health services.

Audit activities in occupational therapy

Multi-professional clinical audit

Multi-professional activity, particularly between occupational therapists and physiotherapists, provides a consistent approach to goal setting and retraining of motor function for rehabilitation of stroke patients Eakin (1991). Such cooperation helps in the drive towards multi-professional audit as well as achieving comparable outcome data on stroke patients. One approach under development is the Assessment of Motor and Process Skills system for evaluating the effect of therapy on motor and cognitive skills (Harvey in Farrer *et al.* 1994).

Outcome measurement

Many audit projects in occupational therapy refer to process measurement (Urry and Grisbrooke 1990; Gleeson *et al.* 1991) but there is now also concern to develop valid, reliable and relevant outcome indicators that measure change in functional ability (Collin 1991). Work on outcome measures has gained momentum although progress is delayed when measures devised in North America must be adapted for the UK (Jeffrey 1993).

Given that occupational therapists are concerned with helping physically and mentally ill people to reach maximum independence in all aspects of daily life, measures of activities of daily living (ADL) are an important part of assessment in occupational therapy and many activities of daily living scales exist (Law and Letts 1989; Dellarosa *et al.* 1991; Intagliata and Sullivan 1991; Friedman and Leong 1992; Fisher 1993; Shah and Cooper 1993). Results, however, are not easily comparable.

One valued measure for occupational therapy is Goal Attainment Scaling (GAS), which provides a feasible, valid and quantifiable rehabilitation assessment method (Zweber and Malec 1990). It is considered to be a sensitive discriminator for evaluating clinical change over time and is much superior to anecdotal and subjective clinical evaluations (Ottenbacker and Cusick 1993).

Small-scale initiatives on auditing outcomes in occupational therapy have been published. For example, Ryan *et al.* (1992) surveyed the effectiveness of hospital-based occupational therapy by using five outcome measures (ADLs, community living skills, client activity patterns, health states indicators, discharge destination). Law *et al.* (1989a) used a specific outcome measure, Quality of Upper Extremity Skills Test (QUEST), to measure four dimensions of movement. Their study notes the difficulties encountered when trying to develop outcome measures specific to occupational therapy.

In the US, criteria mapping is regarded as a reliable and flexible audit method that reflects patients' different clinical requirements (Law *et al.* 1989b). These authors argue that a criteria map can be used as a continuous quality monitoring system that reflects the goals of an occupational therapy department. A similarly comprehensive tool has been developed in Canada, the Canadian Outcome Performance Measure (COPM) (Law *et al.* 1991). Objectives are set in negotiation with the patient, who selects which skills are of particular relevance to him/her. At the end of treatment, the patient is reassessed and contributes to the evaluation of the objectives set. This measure is now used in several occupational therapy services in the UK.

More generally, Jeffrey (1993) advocates the World Health Organization's (WHO) classification of impairment, disability and handicap for classifying outcome measures. She argues that medical outcome scales concentrate on impairment and disability only; handicap is neglected, which is of concern to occupational therapists. Wade (1992) describes measures that exist for four identified steps of audit – input, structure, process and outcome – and argues that the most important measures are those related to case-mix and outcome. Measures of case-mix relate to severity and prognosis whereas outcome measures relate to disability.

Audit activities in physiotherapy

Peer review

The professional literature, especially in the US, reflects the importance given to peer review as an audit method. As early as the 1970s it was proposed that patient care audit should be carried out on a peer review basis by an audit review committee (Bromley 1978). More recently, peer review has been seen as a useful mechanism for reviewing outcomes (El-Din 1991) and process with respect to patient assessment and goal setting (Wainwright *et al.* 1992).

Outcome measurement

As in occupational therapy, there is a strong interest in physiotherapy for quality of life measures. Physiotherapy is generally regarded as more amenable to measurement than occupational therapy and standard outcome measures that are reliable, valid, responsive and practical are a feasible area for development (Jette 1993). Mobility scales used as outcome measures are commonly used. We note Squires *et al.*'s (1991) use of a mobility index in establishing outcomes for physiotherapy intervention in a day unit.

As for clinical psychology, patient satisfaction surveys are used in physiotherapy as a measure of outcome (McCallum 1990). The effectiveness and efficiency of physiotherapy treatment has also been measured using QALYs (Quality Adjusted Life Years) but their sensitivity as outcome measures is questioned (Haas 1993).

Structure, process and outcome measurement

Many studies are concerned with the evaluation of the effectiveness of physiotherapy and so cover process as well as outcome (Kaye 1991; Chiodo *et al.* 1992).

For example, a large audit project in an orthopaedic department showed that physiotherapy input has a positive effect on functional outcome for patients undergoing total hip replacement (Gealer and Hackett 1992).

The TELER system (Treatment Evaluation by Le Roux's method) was developed specifically for physiotherapy as part of the National Nursing and Therapy Audit Programme (Department of Health 1994b). It is a tool for clinicians and managers to collect information on the structure and process, as well as the outcome, of their service (Mawson and McCreadie 1993). The system has undergone trials in several health authorities in England.

Audit activities in speech and language therapy

Process measurement

In the late 1970s and 1980s, work on service delivery was undertaken (types of patients seen, their ages, differences in care provision between different districts) (Enderby and Davies 1989; David and Enderby 1990). A survey of the introduction of speech and language therapy assistants in three health districts noted the poor quality of speech and language therapy databases, especially in relation to process measures (Davies and van der Gaag 1992).

Outcome measurement

The knowledge base and the profession's concern for issues relevant to service delivery (e.g. rationing, skill-mix) prepared speech and language therapists for audit activities, which developed in an explicit way from 1990. As early as the 1970s, speech and language therapy started looking at issues of efficacy, particularly in the area of aphasia and other acute fields.

There is a lot of enthusiasm amongst speech and language therapists for outcome evaluation even though few valid outcome measures exist. However, several initiatives are under way, for example, an outcome scale that can be adapted locally and used either in a uni- or multi-professional setting (Enderby 1992). The scale is based on the WHO scale of impairment/disability/handicap, to which the category of distress has been added.

Many local studies into outcome measurement are developing. One example is a project in a rehabilitation department that aims to specify criteria that can predict outcome, influence practice and evaluate intervention (Kirkwood in Farrer *et al.* 1994).

Process and outcome measurement

The Audit and Outcome Project, supported by the Department of Health and completed in 1993, aimed to:

- conduct a pilot study into clinical audit procedures for speech and language therapy services in the UK in three health districts
- identify the principles and practices of audit which could be incorporated into routine clinical practice
- contribute to the formulation of national guidelines on clinical audit methods for speech and language therapy services.

Process and outcome data were analysed against national standards of good practice. The audit guidebook subsequently published contains guidelines for developing process and outcome measures and consumer feedback (CSLT 1993). The guidelines on consumer feedback techniques include questionnaires, individual interviews, access to local community organizations, consumer fora, multi-professional peer review and quality circles. The outcome measures proposed belong to the two broad categories of satisfaction questionnaires (from the point of view of users and therapists) and pre- and post-intervention measures that rate the level of change in the client's communication skills. Although written for speech and language therapists, this guidebook is likely to be a useful source of practical knowledge on audit for all health professionals.

Appendix 5
The case study sites

Anémone Kober and Maurice Kogan

This appendix describes briefly the focus of our research and the organizational structures in each of the nine sites.

Site 1

Focus

The focus of our research was on audit in speech and language therapy, occupational therapy and physiotherapy.

Organizational structure of the trust

This was a large first-wave trust, including a teaching hospital. It covered the whole range of acute and community activities other than learning disabilities and ambulance services and employed about 6,000 people.

The trust was organized into clinical directorates, some with sub-directorates. Community services were not separate but 'underpinned all the directorates'.

The trust board included the executive directors: the chief executive, the directors of finance, operations (also nursing adviser) and personnel. They also constituted an executive team. The board had powerful and knowledgeable non-executive directors. It included all 13 clinical directors and their general managers who were said to be jointly responsible for running the directorate, although it seemed that the clinical directors were in charge.

Organization of the professions

Physiotherapy and occupational therapy were divided between the directorates so that each directorate had its own head of service. Speech and language therapy, a smaller discipline, was based only in a couple of directorates. The accountability of the heads of professional services was divided between the clinical directorate or sub-directorate for their services and the director of operations of the trust for professional matters. Each therapy also had a professional adviser, not managerially accountable for therapists but a source of professional advice for the trust and its senior directors.

Development of audit

As required by contract, the chief executive made sure that there was medical audit throughout. However, other forms of clinical audit were practised individually, or sometimes collaboratively, by the other professions without constituting a single planned entity. The emphasis of medical audit was on outcome measures which would give practitioners knowledge about how well they were performing. Also, outcomes enabled purchasers to satisfy themselves about what was happening. Process analysis was not favoured by the chief executive on the grounds that it would mean interference in working discretion and would not prove whether there was any benefit from the inputs.

There was no director of quality. The job of promoting quality was attached to all managerial positions. Medical audit was largely separate. There was no evidence of total quality management or other quality assurance activities.

The impetus for clinical audit had come from an advisory group, at regional level, comprising a representative from six therapy professions. Work undertaken by this group had led to a range of projects at the site. Standards setting and uniprofessional audit was well advanced in physiotherapy, occupational therapy and speech and language therapy. Several multi-professional initiatives were in progress; each were large scale projects tackling a number of complex issues. Links between the professional heads of service and management were weak, which made it difficult to achieve change in areas which required management input.

Site 2

Focus

The focus of our research in this site was on audit in the four therapy professions, with particular emphasis on clinical psychology.

Organizational structure of the trust

The site was a large trust, providing acute and community services. It was headed by the chief executive and six directors who formed the board of managers. The director of contracting and quality had responsibility for therapy services across the trust.

Acute services were organized into nine clinical directorates, each headed by a medical director and a business manager. Community services were organized into six geographical localities, each headed by a locality manager who was responsible for the whole range of services within each locality.

The site had two main external purchasers, the health authority and GP fundholders. Since 1993, the contracting process involved giving responsibility to providers to write their own service specifications and to submit these to the district health authority on a set date for discussion and agreement.

Organization of the professions

A clinical services consortium served all the localities and clinical directorates. It consisted of all the therapy professions (speech and language therapy, physiotherapy, occupational therapy, clinical psychology and others). Each profession had a head of service and the heads met regularly. The professions were managerially linked in the centralized consortium. This arrangement was a relatively recent development. Previously, the professions had been accountable to general managers.

The heads held managerial and professional responsibility across the trust for their profession, through the heads of specialty. Therapists worked within multi-professional clinical teams and were managerially and professionally accountable to the professional head. However, the team manager was responsible for day-to-day management issues.

Development of audit

Audit by the clinical directorates and localities was monitored by the purchasers through annual audit reports and feedback meetings. Purchasers set audit targets for each clinical directorate and locality. Current areas were related to national standards required under the Patient's Charter.

Internal service agreements were in the process of being developed. These would involve the directorates and localities acting as purchasers and the clinical services consortium as a provider. It was expected that quality specifications within the internal service agreements would develop.

Site 3

Focus

The focus of our research was on all four therapy professions, with particular emphasis on the learning disabilities service.

Organizational structure of the unit

The site was a community health unit, currently directly managed by the district health authority. It was to gain trust status in April 1994. The unit itself dated from April 1993, and was the result of a merger between a unit comprising the district therapy services and the community services unit of the city.

A commissioning agency was the major purchaser. This agency also placed contracts with the learning disability service on behalf of other districts in the region. The purchasers were not yet placing requirements for clinical audit in their contracts. However, there were perceptions that the role of purchasers was becoming more important, particularly in the case of GP fund-holders.

Organization of the professions

The professions were working within a matrix structure. They were accountable to the professional managers of the individual therapy services and the directors of the five patient service sectors.

Development of audit

The region was perceived to be experiencing problems as far as audit activities were concerned. Audit support staff had changed their employment and it was difficult for provider units to gain support for audit activities. There was also a feeling that there was no integration at regional level of the various existing quality and audit initiatives.

Clinical audit was essentially uni-professional. Before the merger, an attempt to develop multi-professional activities had taken place in the unit comprising the therapy services. However, these initiatives had been disrupted by the merger. The uncertainty caused by continuous organizational change was felt to have slowed down the development of clinical audit, particularly multi-professional audit. However, audit of uni-professional outcomes was starting to develop particularly in clinical psychology and physiotherapy. At the level of the individual patient, multi-professional case reviews took place, involving all professions and carers. These procedures were being developed into audit standards.

Site 4

Focus

The focus was on audit in the occupational therapy and physiotherapy departments.

Organizational structure of the unit

The unit was a district acute hospital including all services apart from the specialized components that a teaching hospital would have (transplants, neurology services). Organization was along general management lines, with the unit general manager and the general director of finance at the top. At the time of fieldwork (April 1993) the unit was about to become a trust.

The newly appointed chief executive of the trust was in the process of setting a directorate structure along service lines. The main directorates planned were operations, human resources, finance, nursing and medicine. Clinical services were to be based in the operational directorate. Each service (woman and child, medicine and surgery non-clinical support, medicine and surgery clinical support, elderly) would be headed by a service unit manager. Within each service, clinical medical teams would be headed by a medical director.

With the move to trust status, the departments would become services. They would be able to employ staff directly and negotiate contracts with external and internal customers.

The main purchaser of occupational therapy and physiotherapy was the district health authority. The purchaser contracts included a range of approximately 60 quality standards.

Organization of the professions

The occupational therapists and the physiotherapists were accountable to their respective professional service managers, who were themselves accountable to the unit general manager.

Development of audit

In the unit, there was no overall quality assurance framework in place. Clinical audit was not well developed in the services, apart from the occupational therapy and physiotherapy departments.

At the time of fieldwork, the purchaser standards were audited externally by the nursing and quality department, based at the district health authority headquarters. This external service review took place every other year. Also, monitoring of complaints procedures, infection control and waiting lists was carried out by the same department.

Site 5

Focus

The focus of the research was on the audit activities of the speech and language therapy service.

Organizational structure of the trust

The site was a large NHS community trust spreading over 65 sites and employing 3,500 staff. The trust was composed of five care groups (community hospitals, mental health, learning disabilities, children services, elderly and physically disabled).

There were five directors on the trust board forming the executive team (finance, medical services, nursing practice and quality, personnel, child services). Non-executive directors included representatives from the local university.

Purchasers were organized in a health commission and did not, at the time of fieldwork, specifically request clinical audit from the providers. However, monitoring of face-to-face contacts and meeting the standards stated in the Patient's Charter was requested in the contracts.

Organization of the professions

On the whole, the professional service managers were accountable to the relevant care group manager wherein most of their work lay. Therapists in the various care groups were accountable to the professional service manager. There were exceptions to this model, notably occupational therapy and physiotherapy. Occupational therapists were directly accountable to care group managers. Physiotherapy was located in the acute trust and contracted out to provide a service to the community trust.

Development of audit

There was no clear link between the clinical audit initiatives in place and contractual requirements by the purchasers.

Medical audit was felt to be well developed and most of the multi-professional audit activities investigated were led by doctors as part of medical audit.

At the time of fieldwork, there was no overall view from the top on clinical audit, which was left to independent professional initiatives. Of those, audit in the speech and language therapy service was felt to be the most developed. There were plans, however, to transform the medical audit committee in the trust into a clinical audit committee with a broader membership and remit for all clinical audit – including medical – activities.

Site 6

Focus

Our research focused on the audit activities of the clinical psychology service in an inner-city community health unit.

Organizational structure of the unit

The unit was under general management but there were plans to move to trust status in April 1994 or 1995. There was a directorate structure with six directors and one deputy unit general manager, each responsible for a service or group of services. The directorates were finance and information, human resources, nursing, medicine, forensic services, and clinical and operational services. The directorate of clinical and operational services was headed by the deputy unit general manager. There were several divisions under this directorate, organized around the two main purchasing health authorities.

Sixty per cent of the contracts were provided by two main district health authorities. There were also some extra contractual referrals, but on the whole funding came down in a straight line from the region to the districts to the directly managed unit/s. This arrangement was likely to change. An internal contracting system was planned, when the heads of the services would act as providers and the divisional managers as purchasers.

Organization of the professions

The therapists were accountable to their professional heads, who held their own budget. However, it was planned that the therapy professions would become jointly accountable to the divisional managers and the professional heads.

Clinical psychology was composed of four primary care teams, each with a team head, but there were also some special posts not belonging to the teams. The service was headed by a clinical psychologist.

Development of audit

There was no general quality system in place. It was planned that each individual service would have an individual business account and a business plan that would outline the quality objectives of the service. There was a quality council for the mental health unit, whose terms of reference were to develop and monitor initiatives in clinical audit. Senior managers and service heads sat on the council. However, its role and power had declined to the point where it no longer met.

Multi-professional clinical audit at team level was better developed than uni-professional audit. The emphasis on multi-professionality was encouraged by professional and general managers, and purchasers.

In the following paragraphs we describe the main characteristics of the additional three sites we visited.

Site 7

Focus

The focus of the visit was on occupational therapy and clinical psychology in the directorate of rehabilitation and continuing care.

Organizational structure of the trust and of the professions

The site was a large mental health services trust. It offered in-patient, out-patient and community services in a large and geographically dispersed area. The trust employed approximately 2,000 staff.

The trust had a directorate structure. The trust board included the chairman, chief executive, five non-executive directors and ten executive directors, including four from the specialty directorates.

The services were split into four specialty directorates including the directorate of rehabilitation and continuing care.

Development of audit

There was no integrated audit or quality assurance system in place. The service had developed a corporate quality group on which the director of medical audit, a director of nursing quality, a nurse adviser for quality assurance and the associate operations manager sat. However, no one was as yet taking overall responsibility for audit. A quality framework had been set up and each head of service (occupational therapy, clinical psychology, nursing) had been asked for a finite number of statements reflecting optimum level of functioning in their service.

Audit activities at operational management level had specific objectives which were not linked with the objective set by the clinical teams. The initiatives developed so far covered complaints procedures and issues identified through user fora. These were fed back into the management system. There were not many links between clinical audit, other quality initiatives and medical audit.

A programme of external audit was starting in which the whole of the mental health care services would be audited externally by the purchasers. The main purchasers involved in this were the district health authority and the Family Health Services Association.

Site 8

Focus

The focus of the visit was the physiotherapy and occupational therapy department.

Organizational structure of the trust and of the professions

This site was a hospital trust that had recently split off from a larger hospital trust. There was a directorate structure in place. The therapists were closely integrated under the therapy directorate.

Development of audit

The trust had a clinical audit research office which was rather overstretched. However, the therapy directorate had obtained regional funding for their audit work and had been able to employ a clinical audit assistant for a period of one year.

The therapy directorate had an overall quality strategy. A quality group made up of senior occupational therapists and physiotherapists met regularly and each member of the group had one area of responsibility for ensuring the completion of the quality assurance strategy of the directorate.

Site 9

Focus

The focus of the visit was the audit activities of the speech and language therapy service.

Organizational structure of the trust and of speech and language therapy

The site was a community NHS trust.

The speech and language therapy service was part of the marketing and contracts directorate of the trust. The professional service manager was accountable managerially to the director of marketing/contracts.

The service covered four main areas (adult/education/community clinics (paediatrics)/adult learning disabilities). There was a service manager and two heads (adult/paediatrics). The other areas (education/learning disabilities) were headed by a senior therapist.

The main purchaser of speech and language therapy was the district health authority. The service also had contracts with a variety of other purchasers (other trusts, GP fund-holders, local education authority).

Development of audit

There was a core quality steering group chaired by the chairman of the trust. There were ten quality sub-groups in place, of which six were clinical/client-group-focused. These sub-groups were essentially communication/planning groups that fostered commitment to quality.

A quality team was in place. It was planned that it would expand from April 1994 and employ quality facilitators deployed in the field. They would act as a link between therapists and the quality sub-groups. As it existed, the quality team acted as an intermediary between provider and purchasers as well as therapists and general management.

Impetus for clinical audit came from three directions: the professionals, the quality framework and the purchasers.

The clinical audit activities were essentially uni-professional and included the early stage of a project on outcomes. The speech and language therapists were, however, involved in a number of multi-professional audit projects.

References

Bacon, R. and Eltis, W. (1976) *Britain's Economic Problems*. London, Macmillan.

Balogh, R. (1991) *Psychiatric Nursing Audit: A Study of Practice*. Carlisle, Garlands Hospital.

Barriball, K. L., While, A. and Norman, I. J. (1992) 'Continuing professional education for qualified nurses: a review of the literature', *Journal of Advanced Nursing*, 17, 1129–40.

Batchelor, C., Owens, D. J., Read, M. and Bloor, M. (1994) 'Patient satisfaction studies: methodology, management and consumer evaluation', *International Journal of Health Care Quality Assurance*, 7(7), 22–30.

Batstone, G. (1994) 'Organisations gaining benefit from clinical audit', unpublished paper, Clinical Audit Conference, Birmingham.

Beck, A. T., Mendelson, M., Mock, J. and Erbaugh, J. (1961) 'Inventory for measuring depression', *Archives of General Psychiatry*, 4, 56–71.

Bell, L. (1991) 'Quality assurance: the case for user involvement', *Clinical Psychology Forum*, 37, 2–4.

Benner, P. (1984) *From Novice to Expert: Excellence and Power in Clinical Nursing Practice*. Menlo Park, CA, Addison-Wesley.

Berwick, D. M. and Knapp, M. G. (1990) 'Theory and practice for measuring health care quality', in N. O. Graham (ed.) *Quality Assurance in Hospitals*, 2nd edn. Rockville, MA, Aspen.

Bond, S. and Thomas, L. (1992) 'Measuring patients' satisfaction with nursing care', *Journal of Advanced Nursing*, 17, 52–63.

Bowling, A. (1991) *Measuring Health: A Review of Quality of Life Measurement Scales*. Milton Keynes, Open University Press.

Bradburn, N. M. (1969) *The Structure of Psychological Well-being*. Chicago, Aldine.

Bradshaw, J. (1972) Taxonomy of Social Need, in G. McLachlan (ed.) *Problems and Progress in Medical Care*, no. 7. Oxford, Oxford University Press.

British Association of Occupational Therapists (1990) *Code of Professional Conduct*. London, BAOT.

British Psychological Society, Service Development Sub-committee Working Party on Quality Assurance, BPS Division of Clinical Psychology (1989) *Quality Issues in Clinical Psychology*. Leicester, BPS.

British Psychological Society, Division of Clinical Psychology (1990) *Guidelines for the Professional Practice of Clinical Psychology*. Leicester, BPS.

Bromley, A. (1978) 'The patient care audit', *Physiotherapy*, 64(9), 270–71.

Brunning, H. (1992) 'Auditing one's work – what do clients think about therapy?', *Clinical Psychology Forum*, 40, 7–10.

Cape, J. D. (1991) 'Quality assurance methods for clinical psychology services', *The Psychologist*, 4, 499–503.

Charlesworth, A. and Wilkin, D. (1982) *Dependency among old people in geriatric wards, psychogeriatric wards and residential homes 1977–1981*. Research Report No. 6. University of Manchester, Psychogeriatric Unit.

Chartered Society of Physiotherapy (1993) *Standards of Physiotherapy Practice*, 2nd edn. London, CSP.

Chartered Society of Physiotherapy (1994) *Quality pack: information on standard setting, audit and outcome measurement for chartered physiotherapists*. London, Professional Affairs Department, CSP.

Chiodo, L., Gerety, M., Mulrow, C., Rhodes, M. and Tuley, M. (1992) 'The impact of physical therapy on nursing home patient outcomes', *Physical Therapy*, 72(3), 168–73.

Clifford, P., Leiper, R., Lavender, T. and Pilling, S. (1992) *Implementing a Quality Review System: the QUARTZ Manual*. Lewisham Hospital, The QUARTZ Project.

College of Occupational Therapists (1989) *Standards of Practice for Occupational Therapy, 1–6*. London, COT.

College of Speech and Language Therapists (1991) *Communicating Quality: Professional Standards for Speech and Language Therapists*. London, CSLT.

College of Speech and Language Therapists (1993) *Audit: a Manual for Speech and Language Therapists*. London, CSLT.

Collin, C. (1991) 'Clinical standards to assist audit in medical rehabilitation', *Health Trends*, 23, 18–20.

Crombie, I. K., Davies, H. T. O., Abraham, S. C. S. and Florey, C. du V. (1993) *The Audit Handbook*. Chichester, John Wiley and Sons.

Crombie, I. K. and Davies, H. T. O. (1993) 'Missing link in the audit cycle', *Quality in Health Care*, 2, 47–8.

Crosby, P. B. (1989) *Let's Talk Quality*. New York, McGraw-Hill.

CSLT, COT, CSP (undated) *Promoting Collaborative Practice*. London, CSLT, COT, CSP.

Dagnan, D. and Fish, A. (1991) 'A satisfaction questionnaire for a child and adolescent psychology service', *Clinical Psychology Forum*, 35, 21–4.

David, R. and Enderby, P. (1990) 'Speech therapy for aphasia operating a rationed service', *Clinical Rehabilitation*, 4, 245–52.

Davies, P. and Kober, A. (1991) 'A methodology for monitoring the health care needs of Oxfordshire', Unpublished article, Oxford Health Authority, Oxford.

Davies, P. and van der Gaag, A. (1992) 'The professional competence of speech therapists. 3: skills and skill mix possibilities', *Clinical Rehabilitation*, 6, 311–23.

Dellarosa, D., San Kuen Chan, R., Pascale Toglia, J. and Finkelstein, N. (1991) 'ADL assessment in acute care: simultaneous grading of physical and verbal levels of assistance', *Occupational Therapy Practice*, 2, 38–45.

Deming, W. E. (1991) *Out of the Crisis*. Cambridge, Cambridge University Press.

Department of Health (1991a) *The Patient's Charter*. London, HMSO.

Department of Health (1991b) *The Health of the Nation: A Consultative Document for Health in England*. London, HMSO.

Department of Health (1991c) *Medical Audit in the Hospital and Community Health Services*. Health Circular HC(91)2. London, DoH.

Department of Health (1992) *Health of the Nation: A Strategy for Health in England*. London, HMSO.

Department of Health (1993) *Clinical Audit: Meeting and Improving Standards in Healthcare*. London, DoH.

Department of Health (1994a) *The Evolution of Clinical Audit*. Leeds, DoH, NHSE.

Department of Health (1994b) *Clinical Audit: 1994/95 and beyond*, Executive letter, (94)20. Leeds, NHSE, DoH.

Department of Health (1994c, but undated) *Clinical Audit in the Nursing and Therapy Professions*. London, DoH.

Department of Health and Social Security (1988) *Hospital Complaints Procedure Act 1985*, Health circular HC(88)37 HN(FP)(88)18. London, DHSS.

Devore Associates (1993) *Manpower planner's guides to data produced as part of the JNPMI Staffing Survey, 1992/1993*. London, Devore Associates.

Donabedian, A (1969) 'Some issues in evaluating the quality of nursing care', *American Journal of Public Health*, 59(10), 1833–6.

Donabedian, A. (1970) 'Patient care evaluation', *Hospitals*, 44(7), 131–6.

Donabedian, A. (1980) *Explorations in Quality Assessment and Monitoring: Volume 1, the Definition of Quality and Approaches to its Assessment*. Ann Arbor, MI, Health Administration Press.

Donabedian, A. (1988a) 'Quality assessment and assurance: unity of purpose, diversity of means', *Inquiry*, 25, 173–92.

Donabedian, A. (1988b) 'The quality of care: how can it be assessed?', *Journal of the American Medical Association*, 260(12), 1743–8.

Donabedian, A. (1988c) 'Quality and cost: choice and responsibilities', *Inquiry*, 25, 90–9.

Donabedian, A. (1993) 'Continuity and change in the quest for quality', *Clinical Performance and Quality Health Care*, 1(1), 9–16.

Eakin, P. (1991) 'Occupational therapy in stroke rehabilitation: implications of research into therapy outcome', *British Journal of Occupational Therapy*, 54(9), 326–8.

El-Din, S. (1991) 'Peer review', *Physiotherapy*, 77(2), 92–4.

Ellis, R. and Whittington, D. (1993) *Quality Assurance in Health Care: A Handbook*. London, Edward Arnold.

Enderby, P. and Davies, P. (1989) 'Communication disorders: planning a service to meet the needs', *British Journal of Disorders of Communication*, 24, 301–31.

Enderby, P. (1992) 'Outcome measures in speech therapy: impairment, disability, handicap and distress', *Health Trends*, 24(2), 61–4.

Enderby, P., Simpson, M. and Wheeler, P. (1992) 'An alphabet of audit', *Therapy Weekly*, 18(25), 6.

Farrer, A., Harvey, J. and Morris, S. (1994) *Audit for the Therapy Professions*, 2nd edn. Keele, Mercia Publications, Keele University.

Feigenbaum, A. V. (1951) *Quality Control*, 1st edn. New York, McGraw-Hill.

Firth-Cozens, J. (1993) *Audit in Mental Health Services*. Hove, East Sussex, Lawrence Erlbaum Associates.

Fisher, W. (1993) 'Measurement-related problems in functional assessment', *American Journal of Occupational Therapy*, 47(4), 331–38.

Fitzpatrick, R. (1991a) 'Surveys of patient satisfaction I: important general considerations', *British Medical Journal*, 302, 888–9.

Fitzpatrick, R. (1991b) 'Surveys of patient satisfaction II: designing a questionnaire and conducting a survey', *British Medical Journal*, 302, 1129–32.

Fitzpatrick, R. and Dunnell, K. (1992) 'Measuring outcomes in health care', in E. Beck, S. Lonsdale, S. Newman and D. Patterson (eds) *In the Best of Health? The Status and Future of Health Care in the UK*. London, Chapman and Hall.

Flynn, N. (1990) *Public Sector Management*. Hemel Hempstead, Harvester Wheatsheaf.

Flynn, R. (1992) *Structures of Control in Health Management*. London, Routledge.

Fonagy, P. and Hignitt, A. (1989) 'Evaluating the performance of departments of psychotherapy', *Psychoanalytic Psychotherapy*, 4(2), 121–53.

Freeling, P. and Burton, R. (1986) 'Performance review in peer groups', in D. A. Pendleton, T. P. C. Schofield and M. Marinker (eds), *In Pursuit of Quality*. London, Royal College of General Practitioners.

Friedman, P. J. and Leong, L. (1992) 'The Rivermead Perceptual Assessment Battery in acute stroke', *British Journal of Occupational Therapy*, 55(6), 233–7.

Gamble, A. (1988) *The Free Economy and the Strong State*. London, Macmillan.

Gealer, J., Hackett, V. (1992) 'How do you measure up?', *Therapy Weekly*, September 3, 4.

Gleeson, R., Chant, A. M., Cusick, A., Dickson, N. and Hodgers, E. (1991) 'Non-compliance with occupational therapy outpatient attendance: a quality assurance study', *Australian Journal of Occupational Therapy*, 38(2), 55–61.

Glennerster, H., Power, A. and Travers, T. (1991) 'A new era for social policy', *Journal of Social Policy*, 20(3), 389–414.

Goldberg, D. P. (1978) *Manual of the General Health Questionnaire*. Windsor, NFER-Nelson.

Haas, M. (1993) 'Evaluation of physiotherapy using cost-utility analysis', *Australian Physiotherapy*, 39(3), 211–17.

Halstead, J., Agnew, R., Barkham, M., Harrington, V., Culverwell, A. and Shapiro, D. (1990) 'The MRC/NHS Collaborative Psychotherapy Project: intensive psychotherapy research in normal clinical practice', *Clinical Psychology Forum*, 26, 30–2.

Ham, C. (1992) *Health Policy in Britain*. London, Macmillan.

Harrison, A. (1992) *Auditing Audit*. Hermitage, Policy Journals.

Harrison, S., Hunter, D., Marroch, G. and Pollitt, C. (1992) *Just Managing: Power and Culture in the National Health Service*. London, Macmillan.

Harvey, G. (1991) 'An evaluation of approaches to assessing the quality of nursing care using (predetermined) quality assurance tools', *Journal of Advanced Nursing*, 16, 277–86.

Hegyvary, S. T. and Haussman, R. K. D. (1976) 'Correlates of the quality of nursing care', *Journal of Nursing Administration*, 6(9), 22–7.

Henderson, S., Duncan Jones, P. and Byrne, D. G. (1980) 'Measuring social relationships: the Interview Schedule for Social Interaction', *Psychological Medicine*, 10, 723–34.

Henkel, M., Kogan, M., Packwood, T., Whitaker, T. and Youll, P. (1989) *The Health Advisory Service*. London, King Edward's Hospital Fund for London.

Henkel, M. (1991) *Government, Evaluation and Change*. London, Jessica Kingsley.

Hoyle, E. (1981) *The Process of Management*. Milton Keynes, Open University.

Hunt, J. (undated) *Quality assurance and nursing*, Quality assurance programme information sheet no. 2. London, King's Fund Centre.

Hunt, S. M., McEwen, J. and McKenna, S. P. (1985) *Measuring Health Status*. London, Croom Helm.

Intagliata, S. and Sullivan, B. (1991) 'Development and implementation of the Rehabilitation Institute of Chicago Functional Assessment Scale', *Occupational Therapy Practice*, 2(2), 26–37.

Jeffrey, L. (1993) 'Aspects of selecting outcome measures to demonstrate the effectiveness of comprehensive rehabilitation', *British Journal of Occupational Therapy*, 56(11), 394–400.

Jenkins, K. and Jakes, S. (1991) 'Evaluation and quality assurance by telephone in a district psychology department', *Clinical Psychology Forum*, 37, 34–6.

Jette, A. (1993) 'Using health-related quality of life in physical therapy outcome research', *Physical Therapy*, 73(8), 529–37.

Joss, R., Henkel, M. and Kogan, M. (1994) *An evaluation of total quality management in the National Health Service. Final Report to the Department of Health*. Uxbridge, CEPPP, Brunel University.

Joss, R. and Kogan, M. (1995) *Advancing Quality: Total Quality Management in the National Health Service*. Buckingham, Open University Press.

Juran, J. M. (1974) *Quality Control Handbook*, 3rd edn. New York, McGraw-Hill.

Juran, J. M. (1988) *Juran on Planning for Quality*. New York, The Free Press.

Kaye, S. (1991) 'The value of audit in clinical practice', *Physiotherapy*, 77(10), 705–7.

Kerrison, S., Packwood, T. and Buxton, M. (1993) *Medical Audit: Taking Stock*. London, King's Fund Centre.

Kerrison, S., Packwood, T. and Buxton, M. (1994) *Review of supra-hospital audit in medical specialties*, Research Report No. 16. Uxbridge, Health Economics Research Group, Brunel University.

Klein, R. and O'Higgins, M. (eds) (1985) *The Future of Welfare*. Oxford, Blackwell.

Klein, R. (1993) *The Politics of the National Health Service*. London, Longman.

Larner, S., Marriot, A. and Pickles, A. (1993) 'The effectiveness of behaviour therapy in dementia: a clinical psychology audit', *National Nursing and Therapy Audit Network Bulletin*, spring issue, 13–16.

Law, M. and Letts, L. (1989) 'A critical review of scales of activities of daily living', *American Journal of Occupational Therapy*, 43(8), 522–8.

Law, M., Cadman, P., Rosenbaum, D., Russell, C., DeMatteo, C. and Walter, S. (1989a) 'Evaluation of treatment in occupational therapy. Part 1: methodology issues in conducting clinical trials', *Canadian Journal of Occupational Therapy*, 56(5), 236–41.

Law, M., Ryan, B., Townsend, E. and O'Shea, B. (1989b) 'Criteria mapping: a method of quality assurance', *American Journal of Occupational Therapy*, 43(2), 104–9.

Law, M., Baptiste, S., Casswell-Opzoomer, A., McColl, M. A., Polataijko, H. and Pollock, N. (1991) *Canadian Occupational Performance Measure*. Toronto, Canadian Association of Occupational Therapists Publications Ace.

Le Grand, J. and Bartlett, W. (1993) *Quasi-markets and Social Policy*. London, Macmillan.

Long, A. F., Dixon, P., Hall, R., Carr-Hill, R. A. and Sheldon, T. A. (1993) 'The outcomes agenda: contribution of the UK clearing house on health outcomes', *Quality in Health Care*, 2, 49–52.

Lovelady, L. (1983) 'Strategies for change in organisations: the use of internal consultants', unpublished PhD thesis, University of Salford.

McAuliffe, E. and MacLachlan, M. (1992) 'Consumers' views of mental health services: the good, the bad and some suggestions for improvements', *Clinical Psychology Forum*, September 16–19.

McCaffery, M. and Beebe, A. (1989) *Pain: Clinical Manual for Nursing Practice.* St Louis, MI, C. V. Mosby.

McCallum, N. (1990) 'A survey of the views of elderly out-patients on their physiotherapy treatment', *Physiotherapy*, 76(8), 487–90.

McLean, A., Sims, D., Mangham, I. and Tuffield, D. (1982) *Organizational Development in Transition.* Chichester, Wiley.

McMahon, R. (1989) 'Quality research in acute nursing care', paper delivered to Nursing Research and Quality Conference, Newcastle Health Authority, Newcastle upon Tyne, 21 September.

Management Advisory Service (1989) *National Review of Clinical Psychology.* Cheltenham, MAS, Series Report Digest.

Mangan, S. P. and Griffiths, J. H. (1982) 'Patient satisfaction with community psychiatric nursing: a prospective controlled study', *Journal of Advanced Nursing*, 7, 477–82.

Marritt, C. (1993) 'The growth of audit – a personal perspective', *Network*, 12(Nov), 1–2.

Mason, R., Glover, L., Grahame, P., Marven, M., Cameron, J., Leahy, D. and Oyede, C. (1994) Audit of lithium screening and monitoring, in Department of Health, *Improving Care through Clinical Audit.* Proceedings of a conference on Clinical Care for the Health Care Professions, NEC, Birmingham, 17 February. Leeds, DoH, NHSME.

Mawson, J. and McCreadie, M. (1993) 'TELER – the way forward in clinical audit', *Physiotherapy*, 79(11), 758–61.

Maxwell, R. J. (1984) 'Quality assessment in health', *British Medical Journal*, 288, 1470–2.

Maxwell, R. J. (1992) 'Dimensions of quality revisited: from thought to action', *Quality in Health Care*, 1, 171–7.

Merrall, A., Patel, R. and Taylor, J. (1991) *Audit for the Therapy Professions*, 1st edn. Keele, Mercia Publications, Keele University.

Moores, B. and Thompson, A. G. H. (1986) 'What 1357 hospital in-patients think about aspects of their stay in British acute hospitals', *Journal of Advanced Nursing*, 11(1), 87–102.

Neave, G. (1988) 'On the cultivation of quality, efficiency and enterprise: an overview of recent trends in higher education in western Europe, 1986–1988', *European Journal of Education*, 23(1 and 2), 7–24.

Neugarten, B. L., Havighurst, R. J. and Tobin, S. S. (1961) 'The measurement of life satisfaction', *Journal of Gerontology*, 16, 134–43.

NHS Management Executive (1993) *Clinical Audit in HCHS: Funding for 1994/ 95 and Beyond*, Executive letter (93)104. Leeds, DoH, NHSE.

NHS Management Inquiry (1983) *Griffiths Report.* London, DHSS.

NHS Review Working Paper (1989) *Medical Audit*, Working paper no. 6. London, HMSO.

Normand, C., Ditch, J., Dockrell, J., Finlay, A., Gaskell, G., Henderson, G. and Whittington, D. (1991a) *Clinical audit in professions allied to medicine and related therapy professions*, Summary report. Belfast, Health and Health Care Research Unit, Queen's University.

Normand, C., Ditch, J., Dockrell, J., Finlay, A., Gaskell, G., Henderson, G. and Whittington, D. (1991b) *Clinical audit in professions allied to medicine and related therapy professions*, Report to the Department of Health on a pilot study. Belfast, Health and Health Care Research Unit, Queen's University.

O'Leary, D. S. (1991) 'CQI – a step beyond QA', *Quality Review Bulletin*, 17(1), 4–5.

Ottenbacker, K. and Cusick, A. (1993) 'Discriminative versus evaluative assessment: some observations on goal attainment scaling', *American Journal of Occupational Therapy*, 47(4), 349–54.

Øvretveit, J. (1992) *Therapy Services*. Reading, Harwood Academic Publishers.

Packwood, T. (1991) 'The three faces of medical audit', *Health Service Journal*, 101(5271), 24–6.

Packwood, T., Keen, J. and Buxton, M. (1991) *Hospitals in Transition: the Resource Management Experiment*. Buckingham, Open University Press.

Packwood, T., Keen, J. and Buxton, M. (1992a) 'The audit process and medical organisation', *Quality in Health Care*, 1, 192–6.

Packwood, T., Keen, J. and Buxton, M. (1992b) 'Process and structure: resource management and the development of sub-unit organisational structure', *Health Services Management Research*, 5(1), 66–76.

Packwood, T., Kerrison, S. and Buxton, M. (1994) 'The implementation of medical audit', *Social Policy and Administration*, 28(4), 299–316.

Packwood, T. and Whitaker, T. (1988) *Needs Assessment in post-16 Education*. Lewes, Falmer.

Perkins, R., Hollyman, J. and Serracino, M. (1992) 'Do we measure up? The development of a multidisciplinary quality assurance and audit system in a psychiatric rehabilitation setting', *Health Trends*, 24(2), 56–9.

Pfeffer, N. and Coote, A. (1991) *Is quality good for you? A critical review of quality assurance in welfare services*. London, Institute for Public Policy Research.

Pollitt, C. (1987) 'The quality issue in British and American health policies', *Journal of Public Policy*, 7(1), 71–92.

Pollitt, C. (1990) 'Doing business in the temple: managers and quality assurance in the public services', *Public Administration*, 68(4), 435–52.

Pollitt, C. (1992) The struggle for quality: the case of the NHS, paper presented to the UK Political Studies Association Conference, Belfast, April 7–9.

Pollitt, C. (1993a) 'The politics of medical quality', *Health Services Management Research*, 6(1), 24–34.

Pollitt, C. (1993b) 'The struggle for quality', *Policy and Politics*, 21(3), 161–70.

Raiman, J. (1981) 'Responding to pain', *Nursing*, first series, 31, 1362–5.

Redfern, S., Kogan, M., Kober, A., Norman, I., Robinson, S. and Packwood, T. (1995) *Clinical Audit in Four Health Professions*. Report to the Department of Health, Centre for the Evaluation of Public Policy and Practice, Uxbridge and London: Brunel University and Nursing Research Unit, King's College, London University.

Rein, M. (1983) *From Policy to Practice*. London, Macmillan.

Riordan, J. M. and Mockler, D. (1994) Care programme evaluation and concurrent audit in psychiatry, in Department of Health, *Improving Care through Clinical Audit*. Proceedings of a conference on Clinical Care for the Health Care Professions, NEC, Birmingham, February, Leeds, DoH, NHSME.

Roberts, H. (1990) 'Performance and outcome measures in the health services', in M. Cave, M. Kogan and R. Smith (eds), *Output and Performance Measurement in Government: the State of the Art*. London, Jessica Kingsley.

Robinson, S. (1994) 'Professional development in midwifery: findings from a longitudinal study of midwives' careers', *Nurse Education Today*, 14, 161–76.

Royal College of Nursing Standards of Care Project (1989) *A Framework for Quality: a Patient-centred Approach to Quality Assurance with Healthcare*. London, Royal College of Nursing.

Ryan, B., O'Shea, B. J. and Townsend, E. (1992) 'Large field studies of hospital based services: lessons from occupational therapy', *Canadian Journal of Occupational Therapy*, 59(4), 214–18.

Secretaries of State for Health (1989) *Working for Patients*, Cmnd 555. London, HMSO.

Shah, S. and Cooper, B. (1993) 'Commentary on "a critical evaluation of the Barthel Index"', *British Journal of Occupational Therapy*, 56(2), 70–2.

Shanks, J. and Frater, A. (1993) 'Health status, outcome, and attributability: is a red rose red in the dark?', *Quality in Health Care*, 2, 259–62.

Shaw, C. (1990) *Medical Audit: a Hospital Handbook*. London, King's Fund Centre.

Social Services Committee (1988) *Sixth Report, Session 1987–88, public expenditure on the social services*. London, HMSO.

Squires, A., Rumgay, B. and Perombelom, M. (1991) 'Audit of goal setting by physiotherapists working with elderly patients', *Physiotherapy*, 77(12), 790–5.

Stokes, J. P. (1983) 'Predicting satisfaction with social support from social network structure', *American Journal of Community Psychology*, 48, 981–90.

Thomas, A. (1993) 'Completed process studies of therapy service', *National Nursing and Therapy Audit Newsletter*, 5(summer), 6–9.

Urry, A. and Grisbrooke, J. (1990) 'Study of occupational therapy service provision in a regional neurological centre', *British Journal of Occupational Therapy*, 53(5), 184–6.

Wade, D. (1992) 'Evaluating outcome in stroke rehabilitation', *Scandinavian Journal of Rehabilitation Medicine*, Supplement 26, 97–104.

Wainwright, S., Crandall, G. and Brodovsky, W. (1992) 'Patient care in focus: peer review', *Clinical Management*, 12(5), 30–7.

Walker, A. (1989) 'Community care', in McCarthy, M. (ed.), *The New Politics of Welfare*. London, Macmillan.

Walshe, K. and Coles, J. (1993) *Evaluating Audit: Developing a Framework*. London, CASPE Research.

Ware, J. E. and Sherbourne, K. D. (1992) 'The MOS 36-item short-form health survey (SF-36): I. Conceptual framework and item selection', *Medical Care*, 30(6), 473–83.

Whittington, D. and Finlay, A. (1991) *Clinical Audit in Physiotherapy, Occupational Therapy, Speech Therapy and Clinical Psychology: a Review of the Literature*. University of Ulster, Centre for Health and Social Research.

Wilding, P. (1992) 'The British welfare state: Thatcherism's enduring legacy', *Policy and Politics*, 20(3), 201–12.

Zweber, B. and Malec, J. (1990) 'Goal attainment scaling in post-acute outpatient brain injury rehabilitation', *Occupational Therapy in Health Care*, 7(1), 45–53.

Index

PURCHASING FOR HEALTH
A MULTIDISCIPLINARY INTRODUCTION TO THE THEORY AND
PRACTICE OF HEALTH PURCHASING

John Øvretveit

Health purchasing has grown in prominence as a result of health reform in Europe and the USA to become one of the world's biggest industries. People's health increasingly depends on the skills and abilities of health purchasing managers, yet little is known about the subject. Ordinary people are becoming aware of the sums spent in their name by 'faceless bureaucrats', and cannot see what value health purchasers add. Although health purchasing is more than paying bills and contracting services, there is uncertainty about the purpose and future role of purchasing organizations in different health systems.

This first book on the subject views health purchasing – both public and private – as a service industry. It argues that, to survive, purchasers have to be more than agents of cost control and must win public support by shaping technological and service changes to uphold our rights and interests. Purchasers need to use service management methods and organization to improve their services to ordinary people.

This book contributes to the theory and practice of the new management discipline of health purchasing, and to an understanding of health purchasing organizations, both public and private. It examines the purpose and methods of health purchasing as a service industry in a rapidly changing and unique type of market. Although concentrating on public health purchasing in the British National Health Service, the book does so in a way which allows comparisons to be made with purchasing in other countries. It presents practical approaches, concepts, and models which have helped purchasing managers and governing board members to tackle key issues. It draws on experience from a variety of sources including a development programme for seven integrated NHS purchasing agencies and the author's research into health reforms in Europe and the USA.

Contents
Purchasing for health – Purchasing and 'market reform' – Health commissioning: purpose and work – 'Decentralized' or 'locality' purchasing – Justifiable purchasing: rationing, priorities, effectiveness and outcome – Contracting and contracts – Quality in purchasing – Collaboration with local authorities – Developing primary and community health services – Purchasing primary health care and the role of the FHSA – Integrating primary and secondary health purchasing – Purchasing agency organization – The future for health purchasing: financing, competition and values – References – Bibliography – Index.

368pp   0 335 19332 3 (Paperback)   0 335 19333 1 (Hardback)

INFORMATION MANAGEMENT IN HEALTH SERVICES

Justin Keen (ed.)

Health services are set on an inexorable drive for more and better information, and are spending millions of pounds on information technology (IT) in an effort to obtain it. But as the need for information becomes ever more pressing, serious problems have come into focus, ranging from the difficulties of collecting accurate routine data to understanding the role of information in management and clinical processes.

This book seeks to clarify the nature of the problems surrounding information and IT, and point the way to practical solutions. It is divided into three sections: policy overview; views from within the health service; and the views of academic researchers.

Contents

Section 1: Overview: information policy and the market – Hospitals in the market – Information policy in the National Health Service – Section 2: The practitioner perspective – Operational systems – Managing development: developing managers' information management – Clinical management – Nursing management – Contracts: managing the external environment – Section 3: The academic perspective – Information for purchasing – The politics of information – A social science perspective on information systems in the NHS – Information and IT strategy – Evaluation: informing the future, not living in the past – IT futures in the NHS – Index.

Contributors

Brian Bloomfield, Andrew Brooks, Jane Clayton, Rod Coombs, Bob Galliers, Wally Gowing, Mark Harrison, John James, Justin Keen, Andy Kennedy, Rebecca Malby, Margaret Marion, Jenny Owen, James Raftery, Ray Robinson, Mike Smith, Andrew Stevens.

224pp   0 335 19116 9 (Paperback)   0 335 19117 7 (Hardback)